Practical Gynaecological Ultrasound

2nd edition

Edited by

Jane Bates, MPhil, DMU, DCRR

Ultrasound Department
St James's University Hospital, Leeds

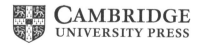
CAMBRIDGE
UNIVERSITY PRESS

CAMBRIDGE
UNIVERSITY PRESS

University Printing House, Cambridge CB2 8BS, United Kingdom

Cambridge University Press is part of the University of Cambridge.

It furthers the University's mission by disseminating knowledge in the pursuit of education, learning and research at the highest international levels of excellence.

www.cambridge.org
Information on this title: www.cambridge.org/9780521674508

© Cambridge University Press 2006

First published 2006
5th printing 2013

A catalogue record for this publication is available from the British Library

ISBN 978-0-521-67450-8 Paperback

Contents

Contributors

Jane Bates MPhil DMU DCRR
Ultrasound Department
St James's University Hospital
Beckett Street
Leeds LS9 7TF

Sean Duffy MD FRCS (Glasg) FRCOG
Academic Department of Obstetrics and Gynaecology
St James's University Hospital
Beckett Street
Leeds LS9 7TF

Tony Evans BSc MSc PhD CEng CPhys
Medical Physics Department
Leeds General Infirmary
Great George Street
Leeds LS1 3EX

Stephen Killick MD FFFP FRCOG
Department of Obstetrics and Gynaecology
Women's and Children's Hospital
Anlaby Road
Hull HU3 2JZ

Chris Kremer MD MRCOG
Pinderfields General Hospital
Aberford Road
Wakefield
WF1 4DG

Hassan Massouh FRCR
Department of Radiology
Frimley Park Hospital
Portsmouth Road
Frimley
Surrey

Josephine M. McHugo FRCR FRCP FRCPCH
Ultrasound Department
Birmingham Women's Hospital
Edgbaston
Birmingham B15 2TG

David W. Pilling MB ChB DCH DMRD FRCR FRCPCH
Department of Radiology
Royal Liverpool Children's Hospital
Eaton Road
Alder Hey
Liverpool L12 2AP

Lynne Rogerson MD MRCOG PG Cert Gynae Ultrasound
Academic Department of Obstetrics and Gynaecology
St James's University Hospital

Beckett Street
Leeds LS9 7TF

Damian J. M. Tolan MBChB MRCP(UK) FRCR
Department of Radiology
St James's University Hospital
Beckett Street
Leeds LS9 7TF

Michael J. Weston MB ChB MRCP FRCR
Department of Radiology
St James's University Hospital
Beckett Street
Leeds LS9 7TF

Itrasound

...provides a fully ...ion to gynaecolo-... ...escribes and explains ...anatomy and physiology, instrumentation and how to make the best use of equipment. Emphasis is placed on how to maximise image quality, and how to recognise normal and pathological features. The volume also assesses other relevant diagnostic techniques and various management strategies, and evaluates the role of ultrasound as part of patient management. It includes chapters on pathology of the uterus, ovaries and adnexae, paediatric and trauma cases, together with management of infertility and other gynaecological perspectives of patient management. Illustrated throughout with numerous high-quality ultrasound images and line drawings, many of them new for this latest edition, this is essential reading for practitioners in training, including radiologists, gynaecologists and sonographers.

With more than 20 years' experience in diagnostic ultrasound, principally as Lead Ultrasound Practitioner at St James's University Hospital, Leeds, **Jane Bates** is well qualified and well known in this field. She is also Past President of the British Medical Ultrasound Society.

Preface

Ultrasound is one of the most important and primary diagnostic tools in gynaecology. Its use continues to increase, and it is now an essential part of the diagnostic process in examining the female pelvis. The increasingly complex technology, whilst producing images of greater detail and diagnostic value, requires a more comprehensive knowledge of ultrasound scanning than ever before. Practitioners must be aware of pitfalls and diagnostic dilemmas, and must know how to produce the best images possible within the capabilities and limitations of their equipment.

Our understanding of physiology and pathological processes and the increasingly successful and minimally invasive treatment options have carved an important niche for the gynaecological ultrasound practitioner. This text aims to provide both a reference for more experienced ultrasound practitioners and a guide and teaching aid for students of ultrasound. Experts from various fields of gynaecology have contributed to the book, to achieve a comprehensive, well-informed and up-to-date project.

The book incorporates both the normal and abnormal pelvis, illustrated with diagrams and high-quality images, together with an emphasis on the role of the scan within the patient's management. It incorporates the latest thinking and practice in various fields, including the acute pelvis, infertility diagnosis and treatment and patient management. The special considerations of the paediatric pelvis merit a separate chapter. Students will find sections on how to make the most of equipment and scanning techniques, in order to maximise the diagnostic potential of their scan.

It has often been said that the greatest hazard of ultrasound is that of the untrained operator. No mere text can be a substitute for practical experience and good training, but this book aims to assist the student in understanding ultrasound and the gynaecological patient. I hope it will also provide the more experienced ultrasound practitioner with an easily accessible and comprehensive reference.

The nature of medical ultrasound is such that developments rapidly outstrip publications. I hope this book will form a basic and enduring foundation which will foster best practice and encourage practitioners to develop their knowledge and skills.

Acknowledgement

My grateful thanks to all the staff of the ultrasound department at St James's Hospital, Leeds.

Equipment selection and instrumentation

Tony Evans

Leeds General Infirmary, Leeds

Equipment selection

Introduction

The selection of equipment for gynaecological ultrasound, as in other clinical areas, amounts to:
- selecting the scanner
- selecting the transducer
- selecting how best to use them

Although the operator may have little or no choice about the scanner to be used, it is important to recognise that it is the combination of all three of the above which is critical. A proficient operator getting the best out of poor equipment is frequently more effective than a poor operator using potentially good equipment in an uninformed, unthinking or poorly thought-out manner. It follows that whoever is using the equipment needs a good understanding of the ultrasonic imaging process, its limitations and characteristics. In particular, there is a need to understand the many compromises that exist, how they come about and how the operator can control the choices being made in order to optimise the quality of the scan. The list below summarises the main considerations to be taken into account before the scan begins:
- spatial resolution
- temporal resolution
- penetration
- contrast resolution
- probe shape and size
- scanning ergonomics

- operating modes (e.g. pulsed and colour Doppler)
- contrast agents
- safety (acoustic, mechanical, electrical, biological, chemical)

Note that the transducer frequency is omitted from the above list. This is partly because manufacturer's probe labelling may be inaccurate but, more importantly, because the probe frequency is not a good predictor of image quality and certainly does not describe it. The operator may well find that a low-frequency probe on one scanner gives a better image than a higher-frequency probe on another.

We will consider each of the features on the list in turn.

Spatial resolution

It is important that small details within a structure or small objects are adequately imaged. This ability may be referred to as the overall 'sharpness' or 'definition' of the image and is described as its spatial resolution. It may be defined more strictly as the ability of the system to identify correctly two targets lying close together. Thus, in Figure 1.1, the targets are sets of pairs of wires lying in a tissue-equivalent phantom and seen in cross-section. In the first case, only the pair in the lowest row are resolved and the other two pairs are blurred or smeared together but, when the wires are imaged using a different machine, the second pair are also resolved, although neither machine can resolve the top pair which are closest together.

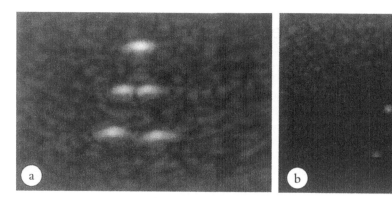

Figure 1.1 Images obtained by scanning wires in a tissue-equivalent phantom. (a) A 3.5-MHz probe is able to resolve the lowest pair (5 mm separation) satisfactorily, the middle pair (2.5 mm) is only just resolvable and the top pair is unresolvable. (b) Using a 7.5-MHz probe all the pairs are adequately demonstrated.

One peculiarity of ultrasound is that the spatial resolution depends not only on the position of the targets in the imaged section but also on the orientation of the targets in that section. One way of describing this is to use the concept of a *resolution cell*. We can imagine the section being imaged as divided into small volumes or cells. If two targets are so small that they fit within the same cell, then they will not be resolved. In other words, details which are small enough to fit entirely within a resolution cell will not be visualised by the scanner. The exact shape of a resolution cell may be complex (typically a little like a flattened sausage!) but it can be described as having three dimensions: an axial length, x, a lateral width, l, and a slice thickness, t (Fig. 1.2). This leads to the need to describe the resolution of an ultrasound scanner in at least three planes and the complication that the three values obtained may not only be very different from each other but may also vary throughout the image. The three values x, l and t are often described as three ultrasound resolutions: *axial, lateral and slice thickness*.

It seems obvious that smaller values of resolution are unambiguously 'better' and this is so, but the means by which smaller values are achieved may involve unacceptable compromise in other features. We first need to consider more carefully what governs each of these resolutions.

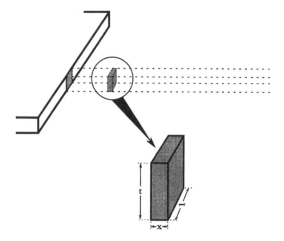

Figure 1.2 The shaded area represents a single resolution cell for the scanning system. Note that the dimensions x, l and t are the resolution values in each direction at the position of the specific cell. Elsewhere, the values may be different.

Axial resolution

The axial resolution, which is the x value of the resolution cell (Fig. 1.2), depends primarily on the pulse length. This is normally a fixed number of cycles (typically 2–3), and so it follows that higher frequencies, which bring shorter wavelengths, will give better axial resolution. For frequencies between 5 and 7 MHz, this will normally be between 0.5 and 1 mm. In almost all cases, it is the smallest and therefore the

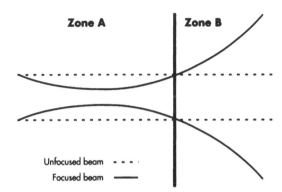

Figure 1.3 The effect of focusing is normally to reduce the lateral beamwidth, *l*, in the region close to the focal zone (zone A). However, away from the focus in zone B, the effect is to degrade the beamwidth and hence also the lateral resolution.

best of the resolutions and consequently, operators are encouraged to make measurements in an axial direction wherever possible.

Lateral resolution

This is the *l* value in Figure 1.2 and is often referred to as the *beamwidth*. Manufacturers use a wide variety of ingenious methods to minimise beamwidth since it manifestly has a profound effect on image quality. In many cases this involves electronic focusing of arrays, which allows the beam to be narrowed only in the plane of the scanning slice and is the reason why the beam cross-section is not circular. Furthermore, the focusing techniques used will often improve the resolution at some depths at the expense of degrading the resolution at others and hence the resolution depends additionally on depth of the target (Figs. 1.3 and 1.4). Manufacturers will often include a figure for lateral resolution in their specification for a probe and with modern equipment working between 5 and 7 MHz it is commonly between 2 and 8 mm. However, this will be a best case and may be quite misleading: the operator is very influential here. Since the focusing depth is normally selected from the scanner's control panel, care should be taken to match the depth selected to that of greatest clinical significance. Many machines now offer the facility for additional focusing on transmission which reduces the beamwidth still further. However, this normally

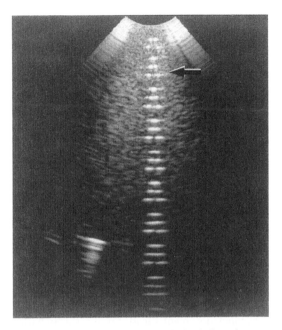

Figure 1.4 Lateral resolution is normally depth-dependent. The region nearest the probe (arrow) has significantly better resolution than at greater depths.

incurs a frame rate penalty and it is the operator who must decide whether the additional resolution gain is worth the price.

Slice thickness

The third dimension of the resolution cell is known as slice thickness and is the *t* value in Figure 1.2. In this case, electronic focusing will have no effect and so it is likely that this resolution will be relatively poor. Some focusing can be achieved by including lenses in the front face of the probe, but this will be at a fixed depth. For electronic probes, this will result in slice thickness resolution in the range 5–10 mm, although for mechanical scanners, the figure will be the same as for lateral resolution since the beam cross-section will be circular. The impact of this clinically is to produce slice thickness artefacts which, for example, will result in transonic areas such as cysts becoming partially filled with echoes which are generated within surrounding tissue. Thus it is important that the operator is aware of the resolution characteristics of the probe in use in order to avoid being misled by such appearances.

Spatial resolution – key points

- The shorter the pulse, the better the axial resolution, i.e. higher frequencies are better
- The narrower the beam, the better the lateral resolution, i.e. in the focal zone of the beam. (Focusing is usually worse at greater depths, with consequent inferior lateral resolution)
- The narrower the slice thickness, the better the resolution. i.e. lenses or curved elements in a plane at right angles to the image

---

Temporal resolution

Temporal resolution is the term often used to describe the ability of the scanner to detect and display rapid movement. Clearly this is associated with the time between samples at a given site, in other words, the *frame rate*. Here we have another compromise involving the operator but based on a fundamental limitation.

The frame rate can be increased by either accepting a reduced number of lines in the image or a reduced imaged depth or both. There are two additional points to note. The first is that if lateral resolution is improved by selecting transmit focusing, this requires more pulses to acquire each scan line. In effect, this is increasing the time per line. Thus the improved resolution must be 'bought' by a reduced frame rate, a reduced depth, a reduced number of lines in the image or some combination of these options. It is the operator who makes these decisions and selects the best compromise, although the control panel of the machine might obscure these stark choices in some cases. For a machine using a sector-shaped field of view, such as a curvilinear array, the compromise might appear as a reduced sector angle, which is a means of reducing the total number of scan lines without sacrificing line density (Fig. 1.5b). Manufacturers of more modern equipment have devised means by which some of these compromises are less critical than was once the case, but the user

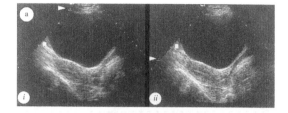
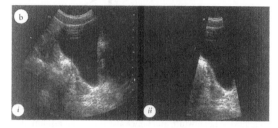
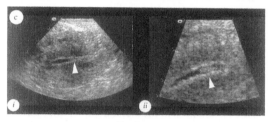
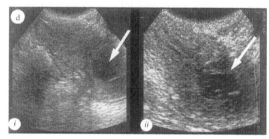

Figure 1.5 Practical image optimisation. (a)(i) The focal zone has been incorrectly placed in the near field. (ii) Correct focal zone placement at the depth of the uterus narrows the beam at this point and results in improved resolution. (b) The longitudinal image of this ovary (i) is improved by narrowing the sector angle (ii), thus increasing the line density. (c)(i) This small endometrial polyp in a patient with postmenopausal bleeding is unclear on the transvaginal scan (arrowhead). (ii) By reducing both the sector angle and depth, increasing the line density, it now becomes apparent. (d)(i) Fluid (arrow) is demonstrated in the endometrial cavity of this postmenopausal patient. (ii) It is better emphasised by adjusting the postprocessing options to improve the contrast resolution.

should watch the displayed value of the frame rate to check how this is working in practice. Gynaecological ultrasound, unlike cardiac or obstetric scanning, does not demand a high frame rate and there is a strong case for using all available means to maximise resolution even if the frame rate drops to around three or four frames per second or less. It is the informed operator who must make this decision.

Temporal resolution – key points

- Depends on the frame rate
- Frame rate is faster when less time is taken to construct the image, i.e. when the image has a small field (in terms of depth and/or width), or is constructed of fewer lines of information, which reduces image quality
- Frame rate is usually of less importance in gynaecological scanning than spatial or contrast resolution and is therefore often sacrificed to improve these latter considerations
- The frequency label on the transducer may not necessarily be a reliable indicator of either the penetration or the resolution capabilities

---

Penetration

The operator will want to be reassured that the equipment selected is capable of producing images down to a clinically acceptable depth. The maximum depth at which useful information can be obtained is determined by many factors, the dominant one of which is tissue attenuation, although it can be increased by one or more of the following:
- reducing the frequency
- using bigger output pulses
- reducing the system noise

The attenuation suffered by the pulse tissue in travelling through the tissue depends only on the frequency of that pulse for a given tissue type. In normal gynaecological practice, this limits 5 MHz ultrasound to a depth range of about 7 cm and 7 MHz ultrasound to about 5 cm. Modern transducer technology does now allow probes to be used well away from their basic resonant frequency (multifrequency probes)

(Fig. 1.5) and this allows the operator to trade off frequency and penetration more explicitly in some cases.

Penetration – key points

- Depends primarily on the attenuation of the pulse, which is less with lower frequencies
- Greater penetration is achieved either by using a lower-frequency transducer or by electronically manipulating the existing resonant frequency
- It also depends on the power setting
- And it depends on the level of system noise or artefact, which can be reduced by using the correct time gain compensation, and is highly operator-dependent

---

Using larger pulses does provide some additional penetration but, because the attenuation is logarithmic, the effect is less than might be expected. Thus a doubling of output power will typically result in an increased penetration at 7 MHz of roughly 5 mm. As we shall see later, there is insufficient evidence to establish firm safety limits at present, and so doubling the power is not immediately vetoed on safety grounds. However, tissue does not behave in a way which might be expected in response to higher outputs and the effect is often to increase non-linear effects and harmonic generation (see section on harmonic imaging, below) which will not improve penetration at all. We therefore conclude that, for the most part, if the probe selected will not provide the penetration required at the highest practical gain levels available, then the operator can only change to a probe at a lower frequency or else find a closer approach to the target of interest.

The most obvious consequence of the high attenuation of overlying tissue has been the introduction of *transvaginal (TV)* probes. Instead of the conventional transabdominal (TA) approach which involves the beam traversing up to 7 cm of tissue, the TV approach will allow many of the key structures to

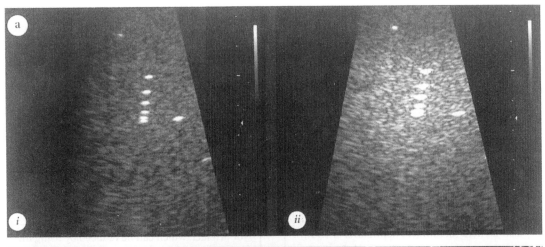

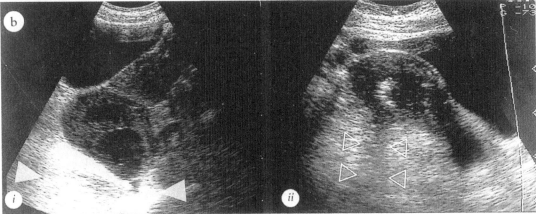

Figure 1.6 Inappropriate time gain compensation (TGC) settings can cause misleading impressions. (a)(i) Correct TGC with good resolution of all the wires. (ii) Inappropriately increased overall gain causes deterioration of both lateral and axial resolution. (b) Acoustic characteristics aid diagnosis: (i) a band of enhancement (arrows) behind this ovarian mass is due to reduced attenuation within the mass, and is indicative of its fluid content (despite the rather solid-looking echoes within it). (ii) The opposite effect of increased attenuation through a calcified fibroid causes posterior shadowing.

be positioned within 2–3 cm of the probe. This allows 7 MHz scanning with its consequent resolution improvement and also allows the operator to avoid other anatomical barriers.

Options for reducing the system noise seem unlikely to provide dramatic improvements in penetration for the foreseeable future. However, the operator has many opportunities to make it worse! Significant image degradation can be caused by misuse of the controls (Fig. 1.6a). If the time gain compensation

(TGC) and other controls are inappropriately set then regions which are generating echoes of an adequate size may not be displayed because the operator has intervened to prevent it. Similarly, the opportunities for creating misleading appearances of either echogenic or transonic regions are many. The operator may also have the opportunity to achieve some noise reduction using frame averaging at the expense of frame rate, although at present the effects are marginal.

Manufacturers may be tempted to declare that their probes are working at a higher frequency than they really are in order to impress a customer with what appears to be extremely high penetration with the tacit assumption that the corresponding resolution gains are available. The user needs to set more store by the actual performance of the probe than by the frequency label.

Contrast resolution
Whereas spatial resolution can be defined as the ability of the system to distinguish two closely spaced targets, the contrast resolution is its ability to distinguish two targets of almost the same nature. In other words, the ability to identify one point or region as being qualitatively different from another solely from the grey levels of the echo displayed from the two. If the echoes generated are in fact different but are assigned the same grey levels by the machine, then the operator will have no way of knowing they are different. In practice, this will always be true to some extent since the range of incoming echo sizes is many times greater than the number of available grey levels in the machine and even when the number of grey levels within the machine is increased, the fundamental limit is set by the number which can be meaningfully displayed by a television monitor and distinguished by the eye. Manufacturers have responded to this by providing a wide range of options for determining which echo amplitudes are translated into which grey levels and most equipment has controls labelled pre- or postprocessing, which allows the operator to choose, although there remains considerable uncertainty about how this can be optimised. The clinical significance of this is illustrated in Figure 1.5d where the same region is scanned at two different grey-scale settings and the diagnostic consequences are clear. Operators should be aware that the 'best' setting will differ between clinical areas and most scanners are set up according to some general compromise. The more sophisticated machines allow the operator to use dedicated set-ups if the machine is dedicated to one clinical area, e.g. gynaecology. How this is determined and validated is problematical.

Contrast resolution – key points

• Depends on the perceived number of grey levels
• By using different processing or set-up options, contrast resolution may be improved over certain relevant regions. However, this will differ according to the tissues under observation

---

Probe shape and size
Transabdominal imaging
The modern ultrasound machine consists of a main viewing and control console to which one or more probes can be attached. The operator on a day-to-day basis may have to choose between three or four probes but at the time of purchase or upgrade, a wider choice will be available.

Linear array This is the most traditional of electronic array formats. It is characterised by being relatively long and narrow, giving a large anterior field of view but requiring good acoustic contact over its whole length. It is not ideal for most gynaecological use because of its large contact area, often referred to as its *footprint*.

Curvilinear array The curvilinear array was developed as a sector version of the linear array and is now the workhorse of many general scanning departments. It has a smaller footprint than the corresponding linear array but is subject to some loss of resolution at the edges of sector towards the larger depths.

Phased array This type of probe has a particularly small footprint because it uses all of the elements in its length all of the time rather than having the active section stepping along the array in sequence. It is most frequently found in cardiology departments where the narrow acoustic window prevents other probe types from being effective. Its main drawback in imaging the pelvis is that its anterior field of view

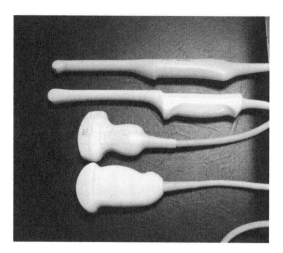

Figure 1.7 Examples of transvaginal (top) and transabdominal (bottom) probes used for gynaecological imaging.

is very limited. In addition it is particularly prone to sidelobe artefacts because of its scanning action.

Thus it is probable that some form of electronic array will be the normal probe of choice for gynaecological imaging. The majority of patients will be satisfactorily imaged using 5-MHz probes, although a small number of difficult or obese cases will only be properly imaged at a lower frequency. In some cases, a higher frequency such as 7.5 MHz will give even better results.

Transvaginal imaging

It is now widely accepted that the optimal images from many gynaecological patients will be obtained using a TV rather than TA technique. The probes developed for this purpose can almost always be fitted directly on to the console of standard machine. Indeed, a number of small portable scanners are now available with TV probes as an option. The range of probe types, shapes and sizes is surprisingly large and there is a marked lack of standardisation (Fig. 1.7 and *see* Fig. 2.7). Potential purchasers would do well to check the viewing angle of a TV probe and be aware of the compromises in resolution and frame

rate which can be associated with working with wide angles.

Scanning ergonomics

The choice of probes and consoles is not entirely objective and operator preferences continue to be important. Having all the controls within easy reach is critical but there are those who prefer more adjustments and those who wish to minimise the number of knobs. There are variations in the weight of probes, the use of foot pedals, the arrangements for caliper measurements and hard copy, the choice of slider controls or others for TGC and the difficulty or ease with which probes can be interchanged. In addition, consideration must be given to whether portability is important. Even the largest machines should be moveable with good wheel design, but there are many small, light-weight, inexpensive scanners available now which can easily be picked up and carried around. The compromise in this case is between portability and image quality and facilities.

Operating modes

The normal operating mode of a conventional diagnostic ultrasound scanner is real-time B-mode. In addition, there may be an option of using a mode called harmonic imaging, which is described below.

Harmonic imaging

It is a feature of soft tissue (and indeed many materials) that as the pulse travels through them it suffers distortion. One aspect of this is the generation of additional frequencies which were not present in the original pulse when it set out. It turns out that if the original pulse was at a frequency f, then the 'extra' frequencies will be at multiples of f. In other words, frequencies $2f$, $3f$, $4f$ etc. will be generated and these are known as harmonics of f. When harmonic imaging mode is selected, the scanner 'tunes in' to one of these higher frequencies (usually $2f$) when it is receiving rather than looking for echoes at the same frequency as it sent out. Since the resolution normally improves with increasing frequency, it might be expected that this would improve the image quality, and in many cases it does. However there is another, more important bonus. Much of the artefact such as reverberation which obscures the ultrasound image is from echoes which do not contain a significant amount of harmonic. By tuning the receiver to the harmonic frequency, these artefacts are partially suppressed. The net result is a sharper and clearer image.

Of course, this will not improve all scanning on every occasion, but there are situations where it makes a significant difference. Some manufacturers offer transducers which can be used in harmonic mode if extra software is bought and hence the machine can be readily upgraded. In other cases, especially if the machine is relatively small and portable, this may not be an option and so purchasers need to consider carefully what their needs really are.

Doppler

For the detection, assessment and measurement of flow, one of the various Doppler modes should be considered. They can be categorised as follows:

- continuous-wave (CW) Doppler
- pulsed Doppler
- colour flow Doppler
- power Doppler

CW Doppler In CW Doppler it is necessary to have separate transducers for transmission and reception, although both can be incorporated into a single housing.

The main problems with CW Doppler are:

- There is uncertainty about the anatomical position of the origin of the signals
- It is difficult to use since, unless the probe is positioned correctly, there may be no signal at all and the operator may not know where to look.
- The angle dependence (Cos θ term) implies that if the vessel is approached at or close to 90°, no Doppler shift will result
- Other nearby moving structures, such as vessel walls, may generate much larger Doppler signals, obscuring those of interest

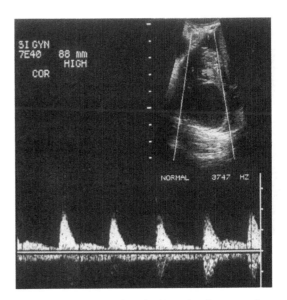

Figure 1.8 The sample volume has been placed over a small artery within this ovarian mass. The resulting spectrum from the artery is displayed as a high-resistance waveform.

As a result of the above, the use of CW Doppler in gynaecology is virtually non-existent and will not be discussed further.

Pulsed Doppler The main advantage of pulsed Doppler is that the operator can select the region from which the Doppler information is to be obtained because the use of pulses allows the timing to be used as a marker. The commonest approach is to arrange for a line to be generated on the image along which Doppler signals will be received and then for a small 'sample volume' to be moved along the line by the operator to indicate the precise depth at which the information is required (Fig. 1.8). The display then shows the Doppler spectrum at that depth and hence the technique is also known as *spectral Doppler*.

Electronic arrays can be used for this purpose since individual elements or groups of elements can be made to generate the extended pulses or act as receivers for the Doppler shifted signals. When the appropriate command is given, the display switches

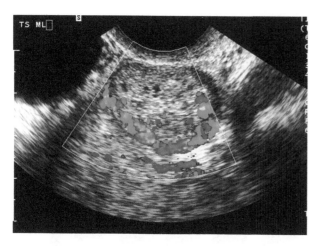

Figure 1.9 The colour box has been located over a mass in the lower uterus, demonstrating vigorous arterial and venous flow around an area of trophoflagtic invasion of a caesarean-section scan.

to the Doppler spectrum which looks much the same as one from a CW system. It is possible using many electronic systems to continue to obtain a live image while the pulsed Doppler information is shown but this inevitably compromises the quality of both.

The spectral trace obtained from a pulsed Doppler system shows an overall pulsatility which is heavily influenced by the downstream impedance. Users wishing to exploit this will want to characterise the shape of this spectral outline and most machines have extensive computerised facilities to allow this.

The main problems with pulsed Doppler are:
- There is a limit to the velocity which can be correctly measured. If the blood velocity exceeds this limit, *aliasing* occurs, which results in the spectrum showing the movement as being in the opposite direction
- Greater depths and higher frequencies lead to reduced velocities before aliasing. Furthermore, if some time is spent in updating the displayed image, then this reduces the maximum still further and hence it is more common for operators to work with recently frozen images of the section of interest

- The operator must select the region to be interrogated by the Doppler beam and only one can be used at any one time. If there is doubt as to whether blood flow is present anywhere in a given region, then this makes searching for it very difficult, if not totally impractical

Colour flow Doppler Colour flow mapping (CFM) Doppler systems superimpose flow information encoded as colours on a real-time grey-scale ultrasound image. With CFM, Doppler information is obtained simultaneously from a large region, possibly even the whole image, allowing the operator to form an immediate impression of the blood flow in the displayed section as a whole (Fig. 1.9). The convention is to use shades of *red* when the net flow is towards the probe and *blue* when it is away from it. The compromise in this case is with the quality and nature of the Doppler information obtained. In order to sample and process signals from the whole section in real time, the complete spectral analysis of the Doppler shifts has to be abandoned. Each scan line is sampled several times (typically eight) in quick succession and the sampled lines are analysed in pairs. A calculation reveals the mean velocities and the uncertainties or spreads are expressed as variances. Thus each small picture element or *pixel* is associated with a single number, which is a mean blood velocity, a positive or negative sign indicating flow direction and a variance value which can be interpreted as a measure of turbulence. The sign determines whether that pixel is red or blue, the mean value is displayed as a shade of the chosen colour and the variance is shown in one of many ways, typically as the addition of some other colour such as yellow or green. It is unfortunate in some ways that the convention is for red and blue to be used as main flow indicators since the ill-informed can misinterpret them as meaning arterial or venous.

Thus CFM systems are very useful for giving a quick indication of the extent of blood flow in a given region but it is important to recognise their limitations:
- The extra time per line carries a penalty in terms of image quality. This may be manifest as a reduced frame rate, resolution degradation or both

- Doppler spectral flow information is lost and hence the facility for evaluating downstream impedance and characterising the waveform is unavailable. It is often necessary to use the CFM as a crude indicator of where to look in more detail using pulsed Doppler
- There is virtually no quantitative information available from CFM systems. Manufacturers use very different methods for determining the colour mapping and most allow the operator to modify it still further. Thus information reported on any one machine is very difficult to interpret and diagnostic markers may well vary between systems
- The angle dependence which limits CW and pulse systems still applies and may lead to confusing artefacts when flow exists but is parallel to the probe face
- The machine has to use some algorithm or rule to determine when the colour information will be allowed to overwrite and hide the grey-scale information. This can lead to missing colour when close to strong stationary targets.

Power Doppler   More recently, some manufacturers have decided to display the Doppler information in a different way, often described as power Doppler. In such systems, all of the power from all of the Doppler-shifted signals within a given region is added together to produce a single value. In this case, no angle correction is needed since no attempt is being made to compute velocities and only one colour is required since there can be no negative power values. The benefit is that a much stronger total signal emerges which does not have angle dependence and allows the identification and display of very small vessels which may be too small to detect with CFM systems. Power spectral Doppler has many trade names, which adds to the confusion, and has mistakenly been described as producing a perfusion map, which is not strictly true. It is closer to being a description of the total energy associated with moving blood in a region and seems to be skewed towards venous flow. Its clinical value, if any, remains to be proven but it is undoubtedly attracting much attention at the present time.

Operating modes – key points

- Predominantly real-time B-mode
- Continuous-wave Doppler not practical in gynaecological scanning because the position of the vessel generating the signal is unknown
- Pulsed-wave Doppler uses long pulses of Doppler from individual elements or small groups within an array. It allows the operator to select a vessel visible on the real-time image and obtain a spectrum.

  The spectrum gives quantitative and qualitative information about the direction, velocity, variance and downstream resistance of the blood film
- Colour flow (CF) Doppler superimposes Doppler information on the real-time image, giving the operator the immediate impression of an organ's vascular 'map'.

  It needs more time per line of information to do this and therefore there are penalties of poorer image quality.

  It gives information on presence or absence of flow and its direction, and an impression of the velocity and variance, but no quantitative information. It is usually, therefore, used in conjunction with a pulsed-wave sepctrum
- Power Doppler superimposes Doppler information on the real-time image as with CF Doppler, but displays only the amout of energy, without any of the directional or variance information. This results in a stronger signal which may potentially identify smaller vessels with slower velocities than CF

Contrast agents

The use of contrast agents is rapidly increasing in all areas of ultrasound. In fact gynaecological applications were among the first to be recognised. There is a wide variety of forms but the common element is that they all contain small gas bubbles. The presence of such bubbles, either in the blood stream or elsewhere, results in a very strong echo being sent back to the transducer. This can result in a vessel or tube being visualised which would otherwise not be seen and hence there can be benefits even in normal B-mode operation. However the interaction with the bubbles can also result in extra harmonic generation and so scanners equipped with this mode of operation might be at an advantage. Furthermore, if the bubble is moving then the echo signal will be Doppler-shifted and so will have the effect of enhancing any of the various Doppler modes as well.

Safety

The safety issues which arise in gynaecological ultrasound can be categorised as follows:

- ultrasonic
- electrical
- microbiological

Ultrasonic

The question of whether diagnostic ultrasound can have harmful effects has been the subject of many papers and discussions since it was first introduced. The reader is referred to the references for a fuller account but it is clear that there is a need for ongoing vigilance in this area. Traditionally the view has been that ultrasound hazards can arise through three mechanisms: cavitation, heating and microstreaming.

Cavitation is the growth, oscillation and possible collapse of bubbles under the influence of the ultrasonic field. This is unlikely in typical gynaecological applications but there is concern where gas-filled contrast agents are employed.

Microstreaming, as the name implies, is the small-scale local circulation of free fluids both inter- and intracellularly and the consequent alterations to cell metabolism.

However, most emphasis is now placed on the thermal effects of ultrasound and the possibility of ultrasound-induced thermal damage. Unfortunately, it is extremely difficult to predict the temperature rise which a given ultrasonic beam would produce in a given volume of tissue and the knowledge that vasodilation would generally occur in most living systems confounds the calculation still further. It is likely that the temperature rise will be related to

the total output power from the transducer and other factors. The situation is complex and rapidly changing. Clinical users therefore need to seek advice and reassurance from responsible expert groups. Such advice is available from the British Medical Ultrasound Society (BMUS),[1] the European Federation of Societies for Ultrasound in Medicine and Biology (EFSUMB) and the World Federation of Ultrasound in Medicine and Biology (WFUMB).

Manufacturers in North America are now required to adopt a system of on-screen labelling[2] to advise the user about the exposure conditions created by the machine at any time and this has now become the de facto standard elsewhere. The system uses two indices, the mechanical index (MI) and the thermal index (TI) to advise users about the worst-case invivo conditions which might arise from their use of the machine in the mode of operation in use at the time. It is for the user then to decide whether or not to proceed.

The MI is concerned about the liklehood that there might be cavitation arising within the tissue being exposed. It is defined as:

$$MI = p/\sqrt{f}$$

where p is the pressure amplitude in MPa after allowing for overlying tissue attenuation and f is the frequency in megahertz. The BMUS advice[1] is that users should strive to keep the MI at 0.3 or below wherever possible.

The TI is defined as:

$$TI = W/W_{deg}$$

where W is the output power and W_{deg} is the power which would lead to a $1°$ rise in temperature in a worst-case scenario. In other words, if the TI is equal to 1, then a worst-case temperature rise of $1°C$ might be expected in vivo.

The ways in which the user might influence the MI and TI values vary between scanners and can be complicated. BMUS and other organisations have drawn up helpful guidance and the reader is referred to their websites for further information.[1]

An additional consideration arises from the possibility of heating directly from the probe itself. In pulsed Doppler mode, the transducer, which has been optimised to produce short imaging pulses, is required to generate and receive longer pulses and its efficiency for this purpose is relatively low. The loss of energy due to inefficiency manifests itself as heat within the probe and there is evidence that, left unattended, in worst-case conditions, some probes can reach up to 60 °C.

Most of the vast bulk of epidemiological evidence supports the assertion that no one anywhere has ever been shown to have been damaged by ultrasonic energy from a diagnostic machine. The epidemiological evidence relating to the safety of ultrasound in obstetric applications has been reviewed on a number of occasions[3] and it is generally assumed that, if the exposure conditions are acceptable for obstetric use, then they will also be reasonable for other applications. Studies have been conducted relating to possible associations of ultrasonic exposure of the fetus with childhood malignancies, neurological maldevelopment, left-handedness and low birth weight. It seems clear that most of the work supports the notion of there being no association of these outcomes with ultrasound exposure. However, they conclude that, on some issues, such as the incidence of left-handedness and low birth weight, no firm conclusions can yet be drawn and hence the recent trend has been towards somewhat more guarded statements than in the past. There is no direct evidence that these effects are harmful but, nonetheless, it should be noted that the general consensus is that most at risk is the developing embryo and that this risk is maximised when the embryo is imaged transvaginally using pulsed Doppler.

It should be stressed that routine clinical scanning of every woman during pregnancy using real-time B-mode imaging is not contraindicated by the evidence currently available from biological investigations and its performance should be left to clinical judgement.

In view of the possibility of ultrasonically induced biological effects within tissues in the path of a Doppler beam, routine examinations of the developing embryo during this particularly sensitive period of organogenesis using pulsed Doppler devices is considered inadvisable at present. It is advisable to minimise output levels and exposure time in pulsed

Doppler mode during fetal examinations and particularly when fetal bone structures lying within the Doppler beam may be preferentially heated.[4]

In this light, it seems clear that the general principle must be to avoid unnecessary ultrasonic exposure of anyone. The use of ultrasound should therefore be to limit the dose to that which is needed to obtain the appropriate clinical information. In other words, it should be governed by the ALARA principle (as low as reasonably achievable), which applies in conventional radiography.

Electrical

Ultrasonic probes in medicine are subject to the same electrical safety requirements as any other electromedical equipment. In the UK, they must satisfy the British Standard BS5724 (or its International Electrotechnical Commission equivalent). This standard is particularly demanding of intracavitary devices such as TV probes since they are in very good electrical contact with the patient. In general, manufacturers are careful to ensure that their equipment complies with these regulations and problems are rare. However, it is important to bear in mind that it is the whole system that must meet the requirements. Thus if the scanner to which a TV probe is attached is itself connected electrically to another piece of equipment such as a camera, video cassette recorder or computer, then the complete system may fail electrical tests even though its individual components have passed. Obviously any physical damage to a probe or its cable such as a crack which might reduce its electrical insulation must be taken seriously, recorded and drawn to the attention of the relevant parties.

Microbiological

While any piece of equipment which is regularly coming into contact with patients must be kept clean to avoid cross-infection, this is particularly important for TV probes. Unlike many other devices used in a similar way, ultrasound probes cannot be autoclaved but some of them have design shapes which make them more difficult to sterilise than others. The considerations include the nature of any cleaning methods, the type of disinfectant to be used, the use of probe covers and the need for an asepctic technique. The issue has been the subject of an advisory statement from the American Institute for Ultrasound in Medicine (AIUM).[5] All such methods must be used in the full awareness of specific advice from the equipment manufacturer since some probe materials will be irreparably damaged by some antiseptics such as gluteraldehyde.

Thus it is clear that this is another situation in which the operator plays the crucial role. By being aware of the situation and adhering closely to published guidelines, the operator can reduce the patient exposure in an ultrasound examination manifold. It has often been claimed that: 'In diagnostic ultrasound, the greatest hazard to the patient is that presented by the untrained or poorly trained operator'.

REFERENCES

1. British Medical Ultrasound Society http://www.bmus.org/safety_of_ultrasoundNF.htm.
2. M. D. Laurel, American Institute of Ultrasound in Medicine/National Electrical Manufacturers Association (AIUM/NEMA), Standard for real-time display of thermal and mechanical acoustic output indices on diagnostic ultrasound equipment, revision 1. AIUM (1998).
3. K. A. Salvesen and S. H. Eik-Ness, Is ultrasound unsound? A review of epidemiological studies of human exposure to ultrasound. *Ultrasound in Obstetrics and Gynecology*, **6** (1995), 293–8.
4. European Federation of Societies for Ultrasound in Medicine and Biology (EFSUMB), Clinical safety statement 1994, Trondheim. *European Journal of Ultrasound*, **2** (1995), 77.
5. S. R. Goldstein, AIUM: report for cleaning and preparation of endocavitary ultrasound transducers between patients. *Ultrasound in Obstetrics and Gynecology*, **7** (1996), 92–4.

Practical use of ultrasound – key points

- The basic gynaecological ultrasound service requires both transabdominal and transvaginal capabilities. It should be subject to regular quality control and safety checks
- Choice of equipment must be informed, taking into account its performance in terms of resolution, penetration and probe selection and design
- The operator must use a combination of both technical ability and clinical knowledge in order to maximise the diagnostic capability. He/she should have undergone recognised training specific to gynaecological ultrasound and maintain regular scanning experience and continuing development in the field
- Good, safe practice includes:
  - regular audit and quality control procedures
  - the use of current guidelines and schemes of work
  - operation in accordance with the ALARA principle (as low as reasonably achievable)
  - recognition of any limitations of the equipment and the technique used

2

Practical equipment operation and technique

Jane Bates

St James's University Hospital, Leeds

Practical approach to image optimisation

Arguably the first consideration in choosing a machine is the quality of the image in terms of resolution. Equipment differs significantly, and should be carefully evaluated before purchase by someone with experience in gynaecological ultrasound. Cost is not necessarily an indicator of quality of image, and in some cases it may be advisable to forgo elements of advanced functionality in favour of a basic, good-quality image.

Intelligent, informed operation of even a basic system is the key to accurate diagnosis. There are a number of controls which can be found on even the most basic systems which, if used correctly, offer significant improvements in image quality which can inform the appropriate patient management. The practical improvements that can be made by the operator to the image are underpinned by an understanding of the theoretical principles outlined in Chapter 1.

As demonstrated in Chapter 1, using the tissue-equivalent phantom, the image should be optimised using the focal zones, frame rate and line density, frequency manipulation and other image-processing options.

Frame rate and line density

The pelvic viscera are usually stationary targets and, as such, can be examined using a relatively low frame rate. This has the effect of increasing the line density with a consequent improvement in diagnostic information (Fig. 2.1).

Focal zone

The focal zone, which corresponds to the area where the beam is narrowest, should be aligned against the structure under examination, e.g. the ovary. When a single focal zone is used it is important to place it to affect the depth of interest (Fig. 2.2). If good resolution is required through a greater depth – for example, when looking at a large, fibroid uterus – the number of focal zones can be increased to three or four. This keeps the beam narrow over a greater depth at the expense, again, of decreasing the frame rate.

Depth/sector angle/zoom

Resolution, in terms of line density, may also be improved by choosing to scan a smaller area. The sector angle may be narrowed when scanning an ovary, for example. For looking at structures in the near or mid-field, the depth may also be reduced (Fig. 2.3). This improves the line density whilst maintaining the frame rate. In addition, small areas may be zoomed for closer examination, achieving a very good line density within a small area.

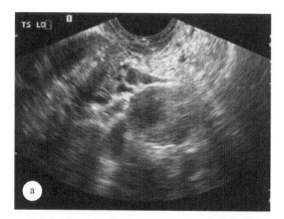

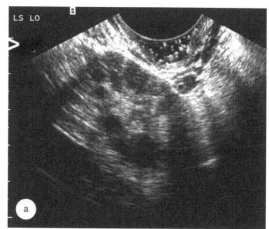

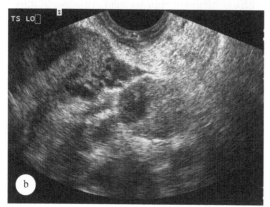

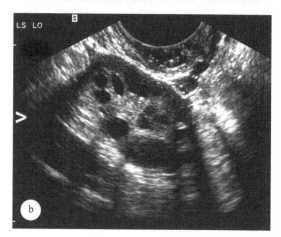

Figure 2.1 Effect of frame rate. (a) A high frame rate reduces the line density, losing image quality. (b) By lowering the frame rate, the line density is increased, giving a much improved image.

Frequency

As we have seen in Chapter 1, the higher the frequency the better the resolution, but the poorer the penetration. The operator must therefore choose the highest frequency possible whilst being able to penetrate to the required depth. Most modern machines with broadband technology allow the user to change the resonant frequency without changing transducers, and the operating frequency can therefore be changed throughout the examination as appropriate (Fig. 2.4).

Figure 2.2 Effect of focal zone. (a) The focal zone is inappropriately placed in the near field, with consequent poor resolution of the ovary. (b) Correctly placed focal zone with good delineation of the ovarian follicles.

Tissue harmonics

The use of non-linear harmonics, if available on your machine, can be very useful in reducing artefacts. In particular, when examining cystic structures, reverberation and noise can often be eliminated, allowing more accurate interpretation of the appearances. Tissue harmonics tends to produce an image which has a reduced dynamic range (looks more 'contrasty')

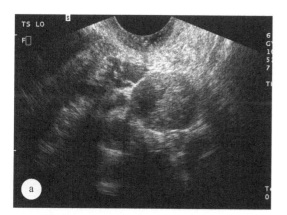

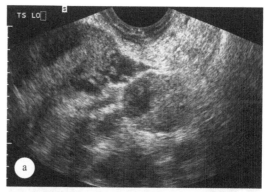

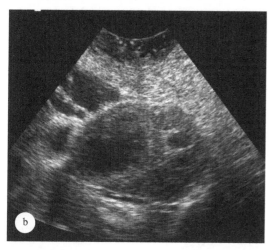

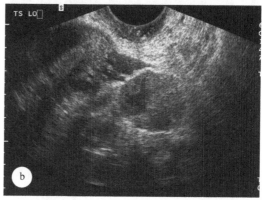

Figure 2.4 Effect of frequency. (a) Transvaginal scan of a normal ovary. (b) The same ovary, using the same probe but switched to a higher resonant frequency: improved detail and resolution, but with slightly poorer penetration.

Figure 2.3 Effect of field of view. (a) Left ovary. (b) Same ovary with a reduced sector angle and depth of field allows a higher line density, and enables the operator to appreciate the ovarian morphology better.

and so is usually used in conjunction with fundamental imaging during the scan (Fig. 2.5).

which could not otherwise be entirely displayed on one image, and can facilitate more accurate measurements (Fig. 2.6).

Extended field of view

Many machines now have the ability to display extended images over a greater field of view. This does not add to the image quality, but can allow the operator to appreciate the extent of large masses,

Choice of approach

The pelvic organs are routinely visualised by two approaches – transabdominal (TA) and transvaginal (TV). Each has its own advantages and limitations and examinations frequently employ both techniques, depending on the reason for referral. Occasionally a transrectal (TR) scan may be useful,

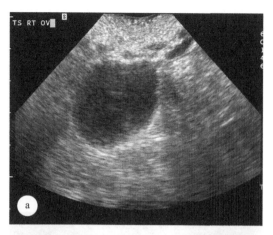

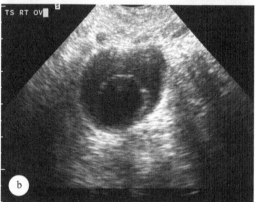

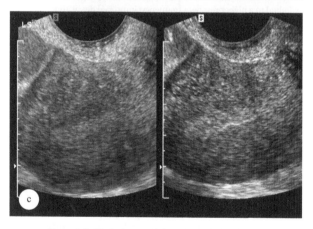

Figure 2.5 Tissue harmonic imaging (THI). (a) The contents of this ovarian cyst are unclear. (b) With THI peripheral blood clot can be demonstrated clearly. (c) The endometrium is more clearly outlined with THI on the right-hand image.

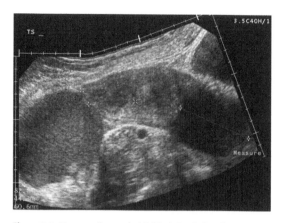

Figure 2.6 The use of extended field of view helps the operator to appreciate the full extent of this case of endometriosis, in which large endometriotic cysts extend well above the fundus of the uterus.

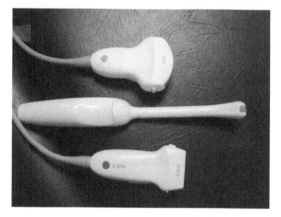

Figure 2.7 Examples of probes suitable for gynaecological ultrasound. Top, curved array for transabdominal scanning; middle, transvaginal probe, bottom, high-frequency linear array suitable for examination of the anterior abdominal wall.

for example, in a postoperative patient with a pelvic collection who is unable to tolerate a TV scan.

Most general gynaecological scanners require at least two probes – a general curved array (around 4–5 MHz) and a higher-frequency transvaginal probe (7.5 MHz) (Fig. 2.7).

The curved array probe is also suitable for scanning other abdominal organs where necessary, such as the kidneys for suspected hydronephrosis, or the

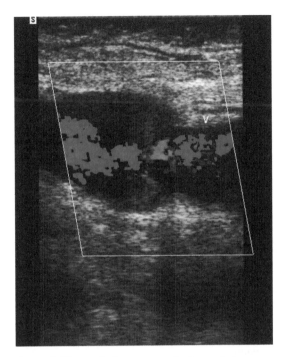

Figure 2.8 The use of a linear array probe demonstrates malignant plaque or 'cake' on the anterior abdominal wall in the near field in a patient with ovarian carcinoma. Note that the plaque is vascular on colour Doppler. As the vessels are approximately perpendicular to the beam, and therefore undetectable by Doppler, the colour box has been 'steered' to create a smaller angle between the beam and the vessels.

liver, spleen and adrenals to exclude metastases in the case of gynaecological cancer. It may also be useful, particularly with ovarian carcinoma, to use a high-frequency linear array probe to examine the abdominal wall for peritoneal or omental plaque from disseminated cancer (Fig. 2.8). This probe has a wide near field of view, with good line density and resolution throughout the depth of view.

Scan preparation

In symptomatic patients who have not had previous scans, it is advisable to prepare the patient for both a TA and TV scan. Women attend with a full bladder, allowing the TA scan to be performed first (see below)

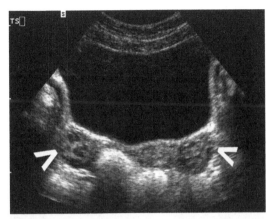

Figure 2.9 The wide field of view of the Transabdominal scan can accommodate the uterus and both ovaries in transverse section.

with the intention of proceeding to a TV scan after micturition.

A careful explanation of the procedure intended and a private scanning environment are essential. It is also good practice to offer the services of a chaperone where possible.

It is invariably necessary first to take a careful history from the patient. This should include the current menstrual state in addition to current and past gynaecological history.

Transabdominal (TA) scanning

The main advantage of TA ultrasound lies in its ability to encompass a comparatively large field of view. This is useful for:

- locating the ovaries in relation to the uterus, particularly those sited laterally (Fig. 2.9).
- demonstrating large masses such as a fibroid uterus, adnexal masses or pelvic collections
- demonstrating iliac fossae, bladder and any associated renal pathology
- demonstrating uterine anomalies, such as bicornuate uterus, which may be more difficult to appreciate on a TV scan.

TA scanning, via a distended bladder, has been used since diagnostic ultrasound began. The full bladder

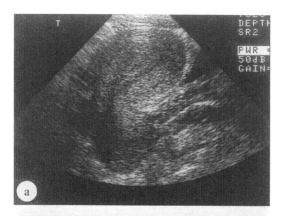

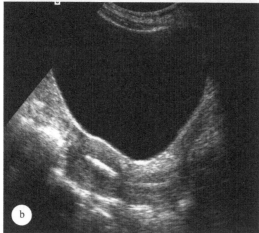

Figure 2.10 Bladder filling on Transabdominal scans. (a) Anteverted uterus with an almost empty bladder. (b) Optimal bladder filling retroflexes the uterus and displaces bowel. Note the strong reflection from the intrauterine contraceptive device.

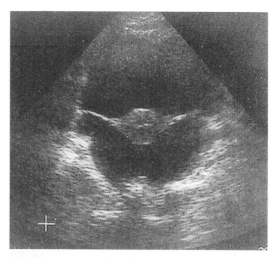

Figure 2.11 The presence of free fluid allows the pelvic viscera to be scanned transabdominally with the bladder empty. The uterus and ligaments are demonstrated.

displaces small bowel away from the pelvic viscera and partially retroflexes the normally anteverted uterus to maintain the endometrial echo at a more perpendicular angle to the beam (Fig. 2.10).

Some patients find the distended bladder uncomfortable, and others are unable to reach the required degree of filling. Associated medical problems, such as incontinence, renal failure or previous bladder surgery, also prevent adequate filling

and TV techniques should be considered for these patients.

The full bladder itself displaces the organs into the far field of the image where the resolution is usually inferior. The bladder can also give rise to unwanted artefacts such as reverberation and mirror-imaging.

Occasionally, ascites may avoid the need for a full bladder, outlining the uterus, ovaries and broad ligament sufficiently to obtain diagnostic information (Fig. 2.11). It is useful, however, to visualise the bladder itself, particularly when bladder pathology is present (Fig. 2.12), or when trying to distinguish pelvic cysts from structures of vesical origin (e.g. bladder diverticula).

Transabdominal technique

The patient is usually scanned supine with the distended bladder as a 'window' to visualise the uterus and ovaries in longitudinal and transverse sections. The uterus is best displayed with its long axis perpendicular to the beam. This varies from patient to patient, in terms of ante- or retroversion and

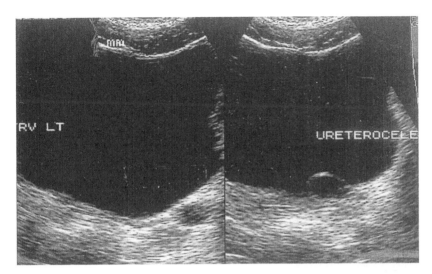

Figure 2.12 Filling the bladder has the advantage of being able to detect other, often unsuspected pathology, such as this ureterocele.

obliquity. Having found the uterine axis, the pelvis can be examined from side to side by a combination of transducer movement and angulation.

The organs should always be examined in two planes where possible, and by turning at right angles to the uterine axis, transverse or axial scans can then be performed through the pelvis, maintaining the beam perpendicular to the endometrial cavity (Figs. 2.13 and 2.14).

The position of the ovaries varies from patient to patient, and according to the degree of bladder-filling. By maintaining the bladder as an acoustic window, the relationship of the ovaries to the uterus can be demonstrated. It is often helpful to identify the ovaries first in transverse section by visualising the uterine cornu and scanning slightly inferior and lateral to this.

It is often advisable to perform any preliminary measurements (of ovarian volume, masses, etc.) at this stage in case visualisation is incomplete or unsuccessful on TV scanning. An ovarian volume estimation requires three measurements truly perpendicular to each other (Fig. 2.15). This is easier to achieve with a TA scan, as the planes obtained TV are slightly oblique.

Transvaginal scanning

The reduced distance between probe and organs in the TV route allows the use of a higher frequency (7.5 MHz). The additional benefit of a lack of layers of subcutaneous tissue (which attenuate the sound in a TA scan) culminates in vastly superior resolution by using a TV technique (Fig. 2.16).

Unfortunately, TV scanning does have some drawbacks: the field of view is smaller, making assessment of larger organs and masses difficult. Large masses will lie outside the transducer's field of view and focal zone, and there is reduced flexibility in the available planes of scan which can make measurements such as ovarian volumes less easy.

The bladder should be empty in order to allow the uterus and ovaries to lie close to the transducer within its focal zone. This often makes the TV scan more acceptable to women than the TA approach.

Acceptability to the patient

Patient acceptability depends almost entirely on the approach by the sonographer and it is rare for patients to decline. The amount of time necessary

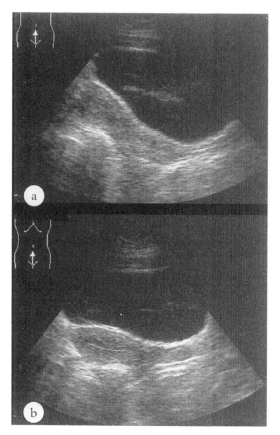

Figure 2.13 (a) The endometrial cavity echo is poorly demonstrated because of its low angle to the beam. (b) With a cephalic angle, maximum reflection from this interface is now obtained. (Note how the echo from the vaginal interface has now disappeared.)

to explain the procedure and put the patient at her ease is always well spent as the benefits of a TV scan in terms of improved acoustic information are enormous.[1] Privacy and dignity must be maintained at all times, and patients may sometimes feel more comfortable with a family member present. There are very few contraindications to vaginal scanning but these include paediatrics and virgi intactae.

Patients may also be offered a chaperone who is, preferably, a female member of staff familiar with departmental practices. This has the advantage of reassuring and assisting the patient whilst also affording a measure of protection to the operator in terms of confirming the nature of the scan subsequently if necessary.

Friendly and professional communication with the patient cannot be stressed too highly, and the majority of litigious cases surrounding TV ultrasound, though few, could possibly have been avoided by employing good communication skills.

Transvaginal technique

The scan is performed with an empty bladder and usually carried out with the patient semi-recumbent, knees bent, buttocks resting on a pad or pillow. This is usually quite sufficient to allow the operator to manoeuvre the probe satisfactorily. (The use of a lithotomy table, with stirrups for the patient's legs, is normally unnecessary but may be found in some specialised departments such as assisted conception units.) Alternatively, the decubitus position, particularly in patients who have difficulty lying supine, is useful.

Using a slightly reverse Trendelenburg position encourages any free fluid to collect in the pouch of Douglas, outlining the posterior uterine wall and, in some cases, the adnexal structures.

In the case of the patient's first attendance, the TV scan will often follow a TA survey, which will have allowed the operator to locate the position and lie of the uterus and ovaries and highlighted any masses. (Patients who attend for follow-up scans or regular screening examinations are usually able to proceed straight to TV scans without first filling the bladder.)

Different scan planes are achieved by a combination of rotation of the probe and angulation (Fig. 2.17). It is sometimes helpful for the learner to imagine the sector beam as a thin fan emerging from, and fixed to the probe, and then retain this mental image as the probe is turned and angled after insertion. As with any scanning technique, it is important to adapt to the individual patient and not perform the procedure simply as a technical process.

The probe is inserted gently into the vagina and may be located in the fornix or withdrawn slightly back down the vagina, to display the uterus fully.

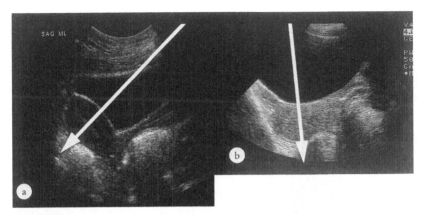

Figure 2.14 Longitudinal sections demonstrating different uterine angles. To obtain a transverse section in which the endometrium is perpendicular to the beam: (a) the best angle for transverse sections is slightly cephalic on this anteverted uterus. (b) This retroverted uterus requires a slightly caudal angle.

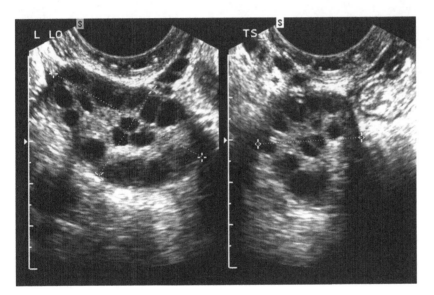

Figure 2.15 Polycystic ovary with measurements appropriate for volume calculation. LO, left ovary longitudinal (left); TS, transverse (right).

Because the field of view is comparatively small, it is necessary to angle the probe, sometimes quite considerably, to interrogate all the necessary structures. Anatomical landmarks such as the internal iliac vessels are useful for locating the ovaries, but it is also valuable to draw upon positional information gained from a previous TA scan if the ovaries are difficult to locate.

Although the problem of attenuation through subcutaneous tissue is avoided by the TV route, large, attenuating masses such as uterine fibroids, and overlying small bowel may obscure vital structures.

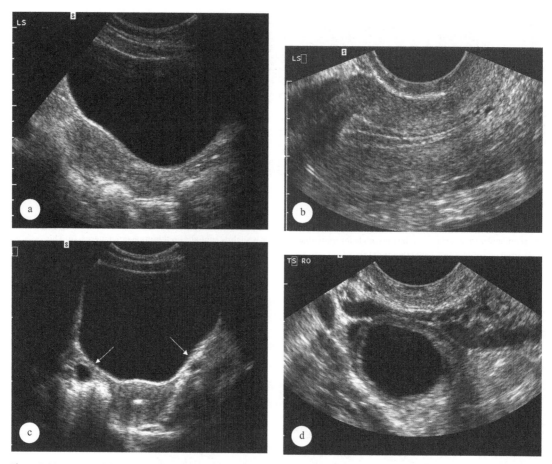

Figure 2.16 (a) Transabdominal uterus. (b) Transvaginal scan of the same uterus as (a), clearly showing the ovulatory stage of the endometrium. (c) Transabdominal scan showing both ovaries. (d) Transvaginal scan of the right ovary in the same patient as (c), showing the corpus luteum clearly.

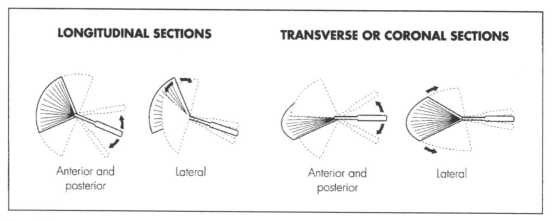

Figure 2.17 Basic transvaginal planes of scan.

This is a particular problem in postmenopausal women when the uterus and ovaries are atrophied. Gentle manipulation of the ovaries and bowel transabdominally with the free hand can overcome this problem and may bring superiorly placed ovaries down into the focal zone of the transducer.

A further advantage of TV scanning is the ability to use the probe to push the pelvic viscera gently and establish whether they move freely over the peritoneal surfaces. Known as the 'sliding organ' sign, this is a useful clue in the diagnosis of adhesions, which will prevent this free organ movement if present.

Manipulation of the transducer by angling, rotating and sliding movements should obviously be gentle and slow to avoid tension and discomfort.

Biological safety

To minimise the risk of infection, the probe should always be covered with a disposable cover. Commercially available condoms are adequate for the purpose of covering the TV probe, but those with spermicidal lubrication should be avoided, particularly in assisted conception units. A small amount of coupling gel should first be introduced into the condom, which is then rolled on to the transducer, smoothing any air bubbles away from the transducer face. Gel is then applied to the outside to maintain contact and facilitate insertion of the probe. Most condoms contain latex, making them unsuitable for use in women with a latex allergy. In such cases, the finger of a latex-free surgical glove makes a useful probe cover.

The sonographer is responsible for minimising the risk of cross-infection and probes should be thoroughly cleaned after each procedure using a disinfectant approved by the manufacturer.[2]

Table 2.1 gives a comparison of TA and TV techniques.

Recognising the acoustic characteristics

It is vital to recognise the acoustic characteristics of organs and masses in order to interpret the scan

Table 2.1 Summary of advantages and limitations of transabdominal and transvaginal techniques

	Transabdominal (TA)	Transvaginal (TV)
Field size	Large: displays relationship of ovaries to uterus	Limited; large masses may be beyond focal zone
	Accommodates large masses within the image	May not be able to accommodate entire uterine section in the field
Flexibility	Easy to examine upper abdomen (e.g. kidneys) with same transducer	Must use TA transducer for upper abdomen
	Bladder and distal ureters can be assessed	Bladder not well seen
Invasive nature	Perceived as non-invasive, so is the technique of choice for paediatrics and others	May be perceived as invasive. Must have good patient–sonographer communication. Privacy essential
Preparation	Full bladder may be uncomfortable or impossible	No preparation required
Resolution	3.5/5 MHz Limited resolution, especially in far field	5/7.5 MHz Considerably superior to TA

correctly (Fig. 2.18). Appearances to be taken into consideration when making a diagnosis include:
- internal echo content and pattern
- margins or capsule of the lesion – well- or ill-defined, focal thickening or nodules
- attenuation characteristics – posterior enhancement, shadowing or mixed attenuation

For example, a simple cyst or follicle should have a well-defined, thin, regular outer capsule, no internal echoes and posterior acoustic enhancement. Any departure from these criteria implies that the lesion is not a simple cyst. Internal echoes with posterior enhancement suggest that the mass is predominantly fluid but contains other material such as haemorrhage.

Recognition of artefact is of particular importance when interpreting the appearances. Reverberation or noise can mimic haemorrhage, pus or even septations. Always ensure you scan from different angles and in different planes to be confident

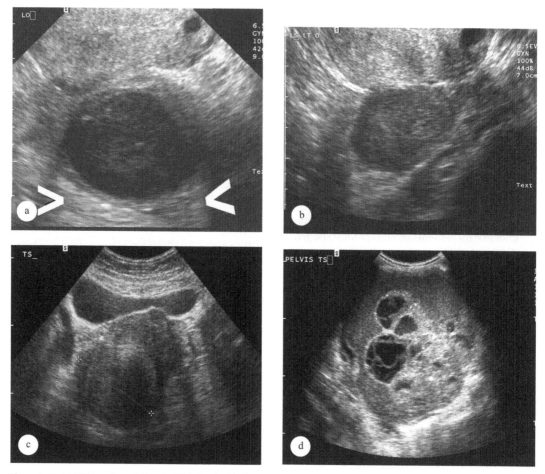

Figure 2.18 (a) This ovarian cyst has a well-defined capsule with a band of posterior acoustic enhancement (arrows). Note the low-level echoes within it from blood. (b) Although this mass also contains low-level echoes, it has no posterior enhancement and is a small, solid fibroma. (c) The fibroid on the right uterine wall is clearly solid, attenuating the beam and making it difficult to demonstrate its posterior margins. (d) Despite the internal echoes, the enhancement posterior to this cystadenocarcinoma demonstrates that it is predominantly fluid in nature.

that appearances represent true findings. Incorrect gain settings can obliterate important characteristics, such as posterior enhancement, shadowing or low-level internal echoes, which would otherwise aid diagnosis.

Doppler techniques

Although colour and spectral Doppler modes are capable of giving haemodynamic information about the pelvic viscera, Doppler often has little to contribute to the general gynaecological ultrasound scan, due to the non-specific nature of the information obtained.

Displaying small vessels within the ovaries is highly dependent on the sensitivity of the equipment, and many normal ovaries appear 'avascular', particularly in the early part of the cycle, simply because the machine cannot detect such small, low-velocity vessels.

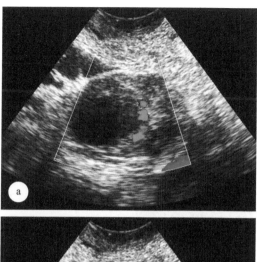

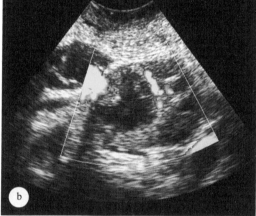

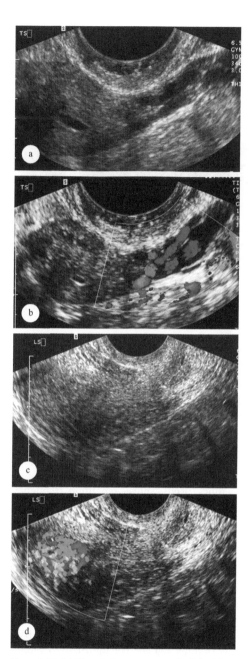

Figure 2.19 Transvaginal section through a normal ovary. (a) With colour Doppler tiny intraovarian blood vessels are demonstrated. Red indicates flow towards, and blue away from the transducer. (b) Power Doppler can be more sensitive than colour, displaying small low-velocity vessels in the ovary.

Power Doppler tends to be more sensitive than colour Doppler, and has the advantage that it is not as angle-dependent, potentially displaying a signal in vessels which are perpendicular to the beam (Fig. 2.19).

The information available from using Doppler is both qualitative (establishing whether something is vascular or not) (Fig. 2.20) and quantitative (measurements of resistance index, for example) (Fig. 2.21). The TV approach, because of its higher

Figure 2.20 (a) The tubular structure on the left of the uterus could be a vessel or dilated tube. (b) Colour Doppler indicates that it is a vein. (c) The endometrium is indistinct in a patient with bleeding following dilatation and curettage. (d) Colour Doppler demonstrates an atriovenous malformation not visible on the grey-scale image.

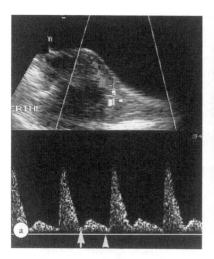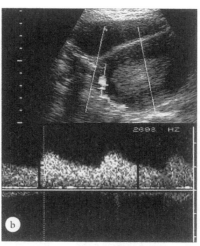

Figure 2.21 (a) The range gate (sample volume) has been placed over a normal right uterine artery. The resulting spectrum gives a characteristically high-resistance waveform with low end-diastolic flow (arrowhead) and a notch (arrow). (b) This uterine artery has an abnormally low resistance (high end-diastolic flow, no notch) in a postmenopausal patient with bleeding from an endometrial carcinoma.

transmitted frequency, provides better resolution with increased sensitivity to low-velocity blood flow particularly relating to smaller intraovarian vessels. Obviously, smaller-diameter vessels with low velocities, such as those within the ovarian stroma, are more difficult to visualise and the ability to demonstrate pelvic vessels depends upon several factors, including:

- the sensitivity of the ultrasound system
- the settings used – pulse repetition frequency (PRF), filter and colour gain
- the transmitted frequency
- the angle of the vessel to the beam
- menstrual stage and state

To demonstrate low-velocity, small intraovarian vessels, the operator should ensure that the settings are as sensitive as possible, using a low PRF or 'scale'. Adjusting the Doppler gain to display the vessels and utilising a low filter so as not to eliminate true but weak Doppler signals. The information gained from spectral Doppler in the pelvis relates to the downstream resistance of the vessel in question. A high downstream resistance, such as that encountered in the iliac vessels and normal uterine vessels (Figs. 2.21 and 2.22), has a pulsatile waveform with

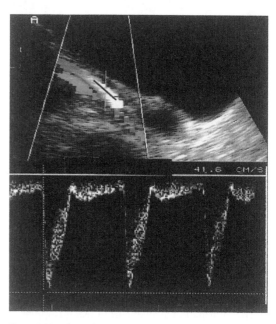

Figure 2.22 The angle corrector has been placed approximately along the direction of flow of this internal iliac artery, giving a peak systolic velocity reading of just over 0.98 m/s.

low end-diastolic flow and often a notch during early diastole. A measure of this resistance to flow can be made by several indices, the most commonly used being:

Resistance index – $\dfrac{A - B}{A}$

Systolic/diastolic index – $\dfrac{A}{B}$

Pulsatility index – $\dfrac{A - B}{\text{mean}}$

where A is peak systolic frequency, and B end-diastolic frequency.

If you are unable to obtain any Doppler flow, check that:

- the angle of insonation of the vessel is low – preferably less than 60° to the beam
- the Doppler gain setting is turned up sufficiently
- the filter is on a low setting
- the system pulse repetition frequency is set for low velocities – (i.e. low 'range' or 'scale' setting)
- the transmitted power is sufficient (within the as low as reasonably achievable (ALARA) principle)
- power Doppler is often more sensitive in demonstrating small, low-velocity vessels

---

Additional techniques

Repeating the pelvic scan after an interval of 1 or 2 weeks can be a useful exercise in some cases; the physiological nature of appearances may be confirmed by scanning during a different stage of the menstrual cycle.

Occasionally, loaded bowel may mimic a mass, or obscure pelvic structures. In such cases a repeat scan after bowel preparation may be necessary.

Saline contrast hysterosonography, in which a small amount of warm saline is introduced via a catheter into the endometrial cavity, improves visualisation of the endometrium and is particularly

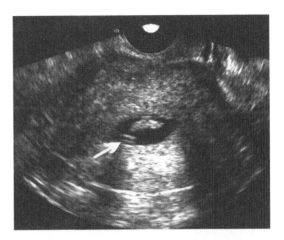

Figure 2.23 Saline infusion hysterosonography. Saline has been infused into the endometrial cavity, outlining this small polyp.

successful in the investigation of postmenopausal bleeding.[3] This has the effect of mildly distending the cavity and increasing the contrast resolution, outlining abnormalities not seen on the routine ultrasound (Fig. 2.23).

The use of contrast media in the investigation of infertility and tubal patency is discussed in subsequent chapters.

Many probes have the option of a biopsy attachment (Fig. 2.24), which enables drainage and biopsy procedures to be carried out with accurate placement of the needle and minimum discomfort to the patient.

The role of the sonographer

Most gynaecological ultrasound in the UK is carried out by sonographer practitioners who have undergone recommended training and assessment programmes in medical ultrasound. It is a well-recognised fact that ultrasound is a highly operator-dependent technique, and one of the greatest hazards in diagnostic ultrasound is not any perceived biological effects on tissues, but its use by untrained personnel.[4]

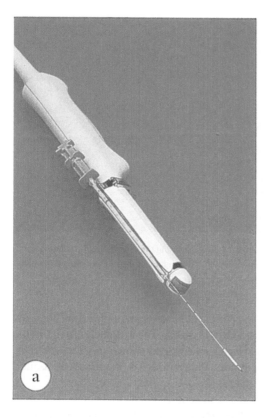

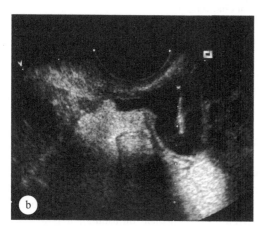

Figure 2.24 (a) A transvaginal probe with a needle-guide attatchment. (The probe cover has been omitted for clarity.) (b) Using the guide, a needle is placed into an ovarian cyst for drainage.

The gynae sonographer is a vital part of the multidisciplinary team, providing expertise in clinical ultrasound techniques and making an invaluable contribution to the management of the gynae patient. Their role in audit and quality control, training, research and development is well established in the UK. Most good departments operate to regularly reviewed ultrasound schemes of work, which outline best practice and provide a framework for monitoring the quality of the service.

The production of images as a record of the examination can provide a useful baseline for subsequent examinations, and can also be invaluable in providing medicolegal proof that the operator has performed a comprehensive examination in a competent fashion.[5] Many departments prefer to store these electronically. Although incurring significant capital costs, this is a subsequently cost-effective system of recording, storing and retrieving patient examinations.

A successful sonographer-based ultrasound service incorporates:

- recognised training
- continuing education
- regular, frequent ultrasound practice
- proper delegation by the medically qualified person in charge
- the use of protocols or schemes of work
- good audit and quality control procedures

Summary

The practitioner should aim to maximise the diagnostic information by:
- carefully assessing the patient's history
- giving a full explanation of the procedure to facilitate cooperation
- utilising the equipment controls properly throughout the scan
- using any additional techniques necessary such as saline infusion

Both TA and TV techniques have their benefits. There are situations in which TA scanning alone cannot deliver the required information – assessing the post-menopausal endometrium, for example, requires the fine detail of TV scanning. Alternatively, large pelvic masses cannot be accommodated in the field of the TV transducer, which may underestimate their extent, and are better appreciated transabdominally.

The strength of the ultrasound examination lies in the fact that it is dynamic. The operator must be both technically skilled and clinically aware, with a flexible approach using a combination of techniques where necessary. Recognised training together with continued professional development will ensure that the scan findings are appropriately interpreted.

Practical use of ultrasound – key points

- The basic gynaecological ultrasound service requires both transabdominal and transvaginal capabilities. Equipment should be subject to regular quality control and safety checks
- Choice of equipment must be informed, taking into account its performance in terms of resolution, penetration, probe selection and design
- The practitioner must use a combination of technical ability and clinical knowledge to maximise the diagnostic capability. He/she should have undergone recognised training specific to gynaecological ultrasound and maintain regular scanning experience and continuing development in the field[6]
- Good, safe practice includes:
  - regular audit and quality control procedures
  - the use of current guidelines and schemes of work
  - operation in accordance with the as low as reasonably achievable (ALARA) principle
  - recognition of any limitations of the equipment and the technique used

---

REFERENCES

1. Royal College of Radiologists, *Intimate Examinations* (London: Royal College of Radiologists, 1998).
2. S. R. Golstein, Report for cleaning and preparation of endocavitary ultrasound transducers between patients. *Ultrasound in Obstetrics and Gynecology*, **7** (1996), 92–4.
3. L. Rogerson, J. Bates, M. Weston and S. Duffy, Outpatient hysteroscopy versus saline infusion hydrosonography (SIH). *British Journal of Obstetrics and Gynaecology*, **109** (2002), 800–4.
4. J. Bates, D. Lindsell and C. Deane, *Extending the Provision of Ultrasound Services in the UK* (London: British Medical Ultrasound Society, 2003).
5. H. B. Meire, Ultrasound-related litigation in obstetrics and gynaecology: the need for defensive scanning. *Ultrasound in Obstetrics and Gynecology*, **7** (1996), 233–5.
6. United Kingdom Association of Sonographers, *Guidelines for Professional Working Standards; Ultrasound Practice* (London: United Kingdom Association of Sonographers, 1996).

3

Anatomy, physiology and ultrasound appearances

Jane Bates

St James's University Hospital, Leeds

Introduction

The female reproductive system comprises the vagina, uterus, ovaries and fallopian tubes. The appearances of these structures on ultrasound depend on the age of the patient and menstrual state and stage at the time of the scan. Throughout the woman's life, particularly during the functional cycle, the organs are subject to physiological changes brought about by the influence of the hormones.

While the main object of the scan in most situations is to examine the reproductive organs, it is also essential to know and recognise other structures within the pelvis, including muscles, blood vessels, ligaments, rectum and sigmoid colon and the bladder and ureters (Figs. 3.1 and 3.2).

Vagina

The vagina is a midline, thin-walled, muscular structure approximately 8–9 cm in length, extending from the uterus to the vestibule (Fig. 3.3). It is H-shaped in cross-section, constructed of longitudinal folds and transverse ridges (rugae) which give it the ability to distend to accommodate the fetus during parturition. In its upper portion, it is contiguous with the uterine cervix and it divides into the fornices – anterior, posterior and right/left lateral.

During transabdominal (TA) scanning the distended bladder, which acts as an acoustic window, does not affect vaginal position. The vagina can therefore be used as an effective landmark, even if the uterus does not occupy its familiar position in the pelvis. The bladder also compresses the vagina, producing the hyperechoic midline echo (Fig. 3.4).

Uterus

The uterus is a pear-shaped, muscular, hollow organ situated in the true pelvis. It usually lies in the midline, anterior to the rectum and posterior to the urinary bladder and is supported by ligaments and muscles (Figs. 3.1 and 3.2). Typical measurements of the adult uterus are 7 cm in length, 4 cm wide and 3 cm in anteroposterior diameter. These measurements all increase in size, on average by 1.2 cm following pregnancy.

The uterus is generally anteverted but may be retroverted or retroflexed (Fig. 3.5). The degree of bladder-filling also has an effect on the flexion of the uterus (see Chapter 2).

The uterus is divided into four parts: (1) fundus; (2) corpus (body); (3) isthmus; and (4) cervix (Fig. 3.6a). Confident delineation of the cervix is not always possible on ultrasound images as there is no clear acoustic difference in the tissues of the body of the uterus and the cervix, unless the cervix is surrounded by fluid (Fig. 3.6b).

The fundus of the uterus refers to the dome-shaped uterine roof, which extends superiorly to the entrance of the fallopian tubes.

The corpus or body is composed of the upper two-thirds and the lower third is the cervix. At the junction

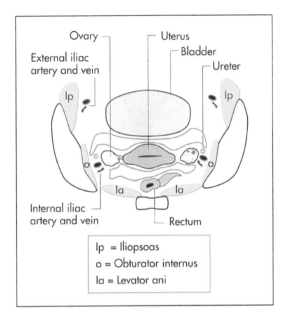

Figure 3.1 Midline sagittal section through the female pelvis.

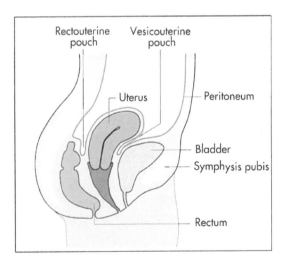

Figure 3.2 Transverse section through the body of the uterus.

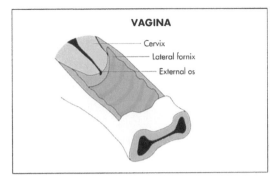

Figure 3.3 The vagina.

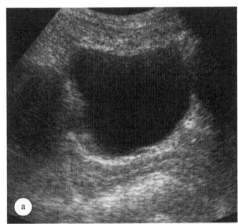

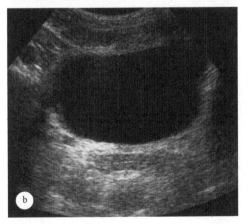

Figure 3.4 (a) Longitudinal section through the vagina. The beam has been angled slightly caudad to demonstrate the echo from the vaginal interface. (b) Transverse section through the vagina.

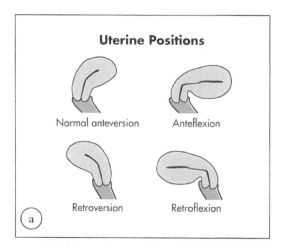

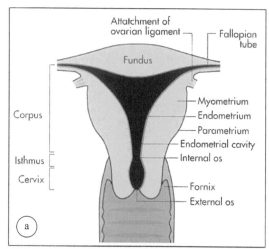

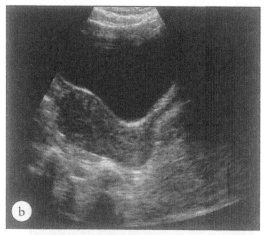

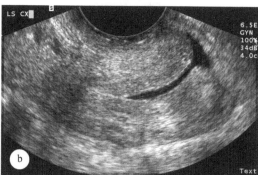

Figure 3.6 (a) The uterus. (b) The cervix is well-delineated on ultrasound when surrounded by fluid.

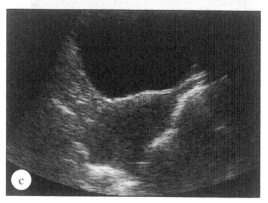

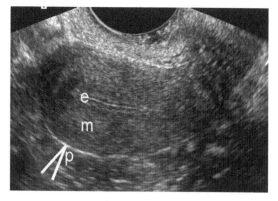

Figure 3.5 (a) Various uterine positions. (b) Normally anteverted and (c) Retroverted uterus.

Figure 3.7 The acoustic properties of the three uterine layers: e, endometrium; m, myometrium; p, parametrium (arrowhead).

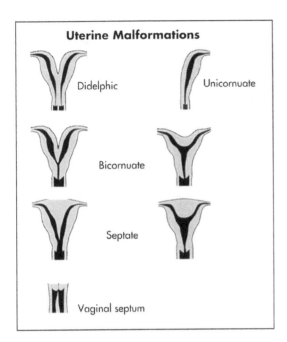

Figure 3.8 Uterine anomalies.

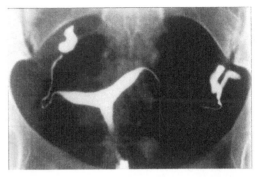

Figure 3.9 Contrast hysterosalpingogram demonstrating a bicornuate uterus. Patent tubes are seen bilaterally with spill of contrast into the peritoneal cavity.

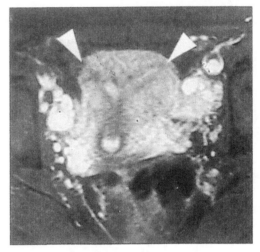

Figure 3.10 Magnetic resonance axial T2-weighted image demonstrating a bicornuate uterus (arrowheads).

of the corpus and the cervix lies the isthmus; it is here that, during the later stages of pregnancy, the lower uterine segment develops.

The two main parts of the uterus have separate functions – the corpus for gestation and the cervix to act as a sphincter.

The uterine wall is composed of three layers: (1) the parametrium – the external layer; (2) the myometrium – the thick muscular layer; and (3) the endometrium – the inner layer. The different tissues of these layers exhibit different acoustic properties (Fig. 3.7). The parametrium, an incomplete covering layer of peritoneum, produces a highly reflective echo outlining the uterus. Lower-level homogeneous echoes are reflected by the thick layer of myometrium and the inner lining, the endometrium, exhibits changing ultrasound appearances throughout the hormonal cycle, giving rise to different thicknesses and reflectivities.

These cyclical changes of the endometrium and ovaries are described in more detail later in this chapter (see Fig. 3.27).

Uterine anomalies

The reproductive organs develop in the embryo from two tubes, the Müllerian ducts. The caudal portions of these ducts eventually fuse to form the uterus, cervix and superior part of the vagina, while the cranial portions remain separate, forming the fallopian tubes. Development takes place from the third or fourth week of gestation and continues into the second trimester. Interruption to this process causes incomplete fusion, which may result in a variety of structural anomalies[1,2] and the more common anomalies are demonstrated in Figure 3.8.

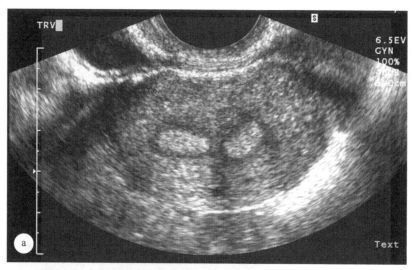

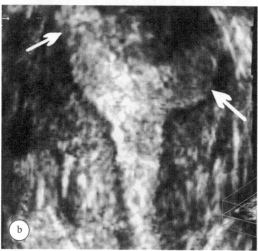

Figure 3.11 (a) Ultrasound demonstration of a bicornuate uterus in transverse section. This may often be more obvious on transabdominal than transvaginal scanning, due to the larger field of view. (b) A three-dimensional transvaginal ultrasound image of a bicornuate uterus.

It may be difficult to demonstrate on ultrasound the more subtle anomalies; these may often be better revealed by laparotomy, laparoscopy or hysterosalpingogram during investigations for infertility or failed pregnancies (Fig. 3.9). Magnetic resonance imaging is also useful for demonstrating uterine anomalies (Fig. 3.10).

The bicornuate uterus is most frequently identified on ultrasound in transverse section, by demonstrating two distinct cornua, each with its endometrial echo, towards the fundus. The advent of three-dimensional ultrasound has also played a useful role in evaluating uterine anomalies (Fig. 3.11) by being able to display the endometrium in coronal section.[3]

Ovaries

The function of the ovaries is to produce a mature ovum every 28 days, to secrete the female hormones, oestrogen and progesterone, which maintain the reproductive cycle, and to support pregnancy.

Table 3.1 Age-related differences in size of the uterus and ovaries

		Infantile	Prepubertal	Reproductive	Postmenopausal
Uterus	Length (cm)	1.5–2	2–5.4	5–12	3.5–6.5
	Width	0.8–1.0	1.0–2.2	4.0	1.2–1.8
	Anteroposterior diameter		1.0	3	1.5–2.0
Ovaries	Volume (cm³)	0.7–3.6	1–6	6–12	<4

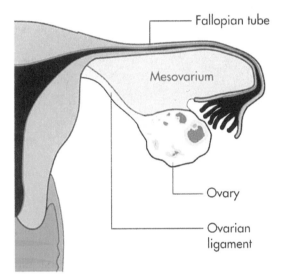

Figure 3.12 Anatomical relations of the ovary.

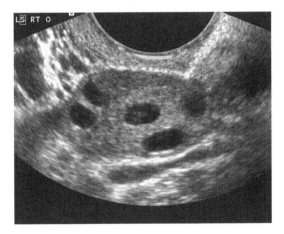

Figure 3.13 Transvaginal scan of the normal ovary demonstrating graafian follicles.

Each ovary usually lies posterior and lateral to either side of the uterus attached to the broad ligaments by its own mesentery, the mesovarium and to the uterus by the ovarian ligament. Its upper surface lies in close proximity to the fimbrial end of the fallopian tube (Fig. 3.12).

Ovaries are oval in shape, usually about the size of a walnut but varying with age (Table 3.1). The ovary is made up of the central portion or medulla and the outer cortex (stroma) within which are contained a number of graafian follicles. It is the follicle which houses the ovum. The blood and lymphatic vessels and nerves are situated in the medulla.

Ultrasonically, the stroma and medulla exhibit quite different appearances: the stroma demonstrates the greater changes during the menstrual cycle. The follicles, a 'soft-marker' for ovarian identification, are visualised in a peripheral arrangement as well-defined echo-free areas in the stroma (Fig. 3.13). Their size varies with the stage of the cycle. The central medulla appears as an area of relatively strong reflectivity with no definite borders.

The mesovarium is mobile, making the exact location of the ovaries variable. The position of the ovaries also varies according to adjacent bowel and the degree of bladder-filling (Fig. 3.14), and may alter position during scanning.[4] This, together with ovarian atrophy following menopause, can make scanning a challenge. It is useful to use ultrasonic landmarks to help with identification. In most cases, the ovary lies in close proximity to the internal iliac artery which can be visualised passing obliquely lateral to the lower third of the uterus (Fig. 3.15). A less easily recognisable but still useful landmark is the position of the levator ani muscle which marks the most

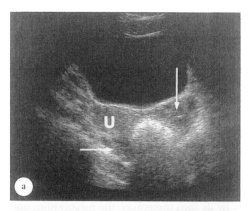

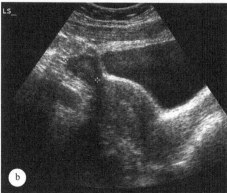

Figure 3.14 (a) Transverse transabdominal scan demonstrating varying ovarian positions (arrows). The right ovary lies behind the uterus (U), (b) Longitudinal section with the left ovary lying above the fundus of the uterus.

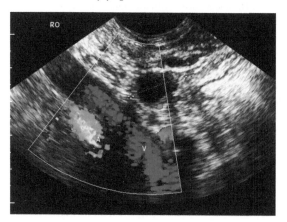

Figure 3.15 Transvaginal longitudinal section through the ovary demonstrating the proximity of the internal iliac artery (A) and internal iliac vein (V).

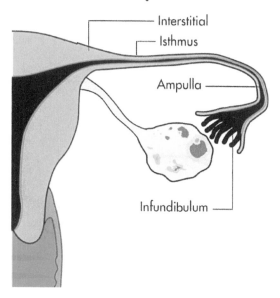

Figure 3.16 The fallopian tube.

inferior position at which the ovary can be located (see section on musculature, below).

For practical scanning purposes, the ovaries can be visualised in a variety of positions from the pouch of Douglas to the superolateral aspect of the uterus.

Fallopian tubes

The two fallopian tubes lie either side of the uterus in the superior portion of the broad ligament (Fig. 3.16). Their walls are composed of the same three layers as the uterus.

Each tube is approximately 10 cm in length and passes laterally, posteriorly and inferiorly from the upper part of the uterus. The uterine opening is minute whilst the abdominal opening, which is in close proximity to the ovary, is larger.

Each tube has four parts:
1. the interstitial portion, which lies within the uterine wall
2. the isthmus – the medial third extending laterally from the upper part of the uterus

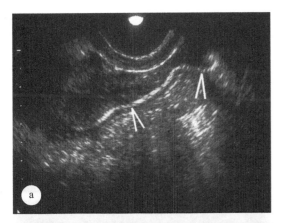

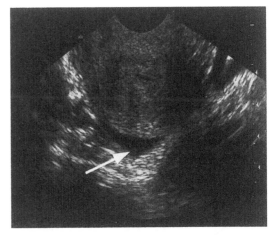

Figure 3.18 Transvaginal axial section through the lower uterus. Fluid in the pouch of Douglas (arrow) is a normal finding mid-cycle.

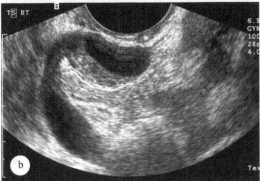

Figure 3.17 (a) Hystero-contrast sonography. The normal (undilated) fallopian tube, not usually visible on ultrasound, can be demonstrated when contrast is introduced, increasing the echogenicity and contrast resolution. (b) The tube is demonstrated when dilated with fluid and debris in the hydrosalpinx.

3. the ampulla, which is the widest part of the tube
4. the infundibulum, which is the dilated funnel-shaped portion close to the ovary

The opening of the infundibulum has tiny projections, known as fimbriae, which serve to guide the ovum into the tube.

The function of each tube is to convey the ovum from the ovary to the uterine cavity. If fertilisation takes place, it usually occurs in the tube.

The normal fallopian tube is difficult to image sonographically as its tiny diameter is beyond the resolution capabilities of most transducers and it is a relatively poor reflector of ultrasound. The over-

all structure may be demonstrated after the introduction of contrast during X-ray hysterosalpingography (Fig. 3.9) or preferably, without incurring the potential hazard of radiation, with hystero-contrast sonograpy or HyCoSy (Fig. 3.17: see Chapter 7). Occasionally, pelvic fluid may be present surrounding the tubes, making at least partial visualisation possible.

Peritoneum and ligaments

The peritoneum surrounds the body of the uterus, forming recesses, or pouches, anteriorly and posteriorly (Figs. 3.1 and 3.2). The anterior recess between the uterus and posterior bladder wall is known as the vesicouterine fossa. The posterior recess lies anterior to the rectum and extends down to the posterior fornix of the vagina. It is known as the rectouterine fossa or pouch of Douglas.

It is not unusual to see fluid in this recess on ultrasound, especially during mid-cycle after ovulation, as this represents a gravity-dependent pocket when the patient lies supine (Fig. 3.18).

The ligaments attaching the uterus within the pelvic cavity are predominantly extensions of the peritoneum in anterior, posterior and lateral directions.[5] The anterior and posterior ligaments

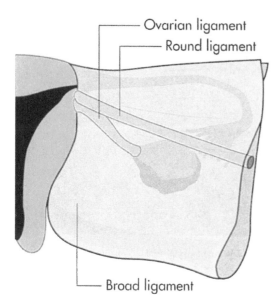

Figure 3.19 The ligaments. The broad ligament is a double fold of peritoneum in which lie the adnexal structures.

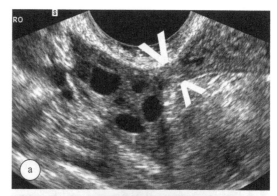

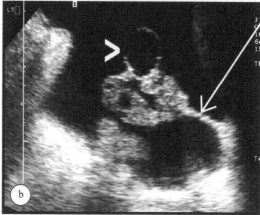

Figure 3.20 (a) Right adnexal area. The superior portion of the broad ligament (arrowheads) containing the ovarian artery. (b) The ovarian liagament (arrow) is demonstrated when surrounded by fluid. A small fimbrial cyst is noted (arrowhead).

form the vesicouterine and rectouterine pouches (see above). Two further peritoneal extensions between the posterior uterine surface and the sacrum form the paired uterosacral ligaments.

The paired broad ligaments are composed of double folds of peritoneum which extend laterally from either side of the uterus to the wall of the bony pelvis. Each ligament contains the fallopian tube in its superior portion, the round ligament, the ovary with its ovarian ligament, blood vessels and nerves (Fig. 3.19).

These ligaments are not easy to see ultrasonically. However with careful scanning in the transaxial plane, superior to the uterine fundus, an arc of low-level homogeneous echoes can be visualised, which represents the broad ligament and its contents as it arises adjacent to the horn of the uterus (Fig. 3.20).

The paired round ligaments are not extensions of the peritoneum, but fibromuscular cords which extend laterally from the region of the uterine cornua and lie within the broad ligament. Each ovary is also attached to the lateral wall of the uterus by the ovarian ligament. When free fluid is present in the

pelvis it is possible to visualise the ovarian ligament as a highly reflective linear echo in the fluid.

Vasculature

The main uterine artery arises from the internal iliac artery. It passes medially, supplying the cervix and ascending the lateral aspect of uterus within the broad ligament. Branches from the main artery further supply the cervix and vagina (Fig. 3.21). The vaginal arteries eventually form the azygos arteries of the vagina as they descend along its surface. These vessels are tortuous and coiled to provide extra length during pregnancy.

The ovary arises from the abdominal aorta, immediately below the renal arteries. At the margin of the

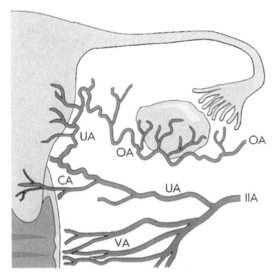

IIA Internal iliac artery   VA Vaginal artery
UA Uterine artery   OA Ovarian artery
CA Coronal artery of the cervix

Figure 3.21 Arterial supply to the uterus and ovary.

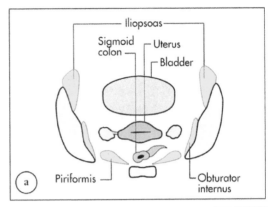

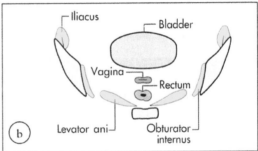

Figure 3.22 The pelvic muscles. (a) Axial section at the level of the body of the uterus. (b) Axial section at the level of the vagina.

pelvis, the artery passes between the folds of the broad ligament. Several of its smaller branches supply the fallopian tubes and anastomose with uterine arteries.

Venous drainage from the uterus is via the internal iliac vein, and from the ovaries is into the venous plexus, from which arise the ovarian veins, lying posterior to the uterus. The right ovarian vein drains into the inferior vena cava, the left ovarian vein into the left renal vein.

Musculature

The pelvic organs are supported by a 'shelf' of muscle on each side. There are four main muscle pairs; the levator ani and the coccygeus make up the pelvic diaphragm. The levator ani lies between the ischial spines and the posterior portion of the pubis and acts as the floor of the pelvis.[5] It supports the pelvic organs and surrounds the rectum, vagina and urethra which pierce it.

The piriformis lies slightly posterior and superior to the coccygeus, and the obturator internus lies against the lateral wall on each side of the pelvis

with the insertion point being the greater trochanter (Fig. 3.22).

The muscles can be demonstrated on ultrasound as well-defined linear structures with low-level homogeneous echoes. Their position is probably most readily appreciated transabdominally, posterior and lateral to the uterus. Occasionally they may be mistaken for pathology, and it is important always to be aware of their location and appearance (Fig. 3.23).

Bladder and ureters

The bladder is a reservoir for urine and occupies the lower portion of the true pelvis anterior to the uterus. The normal full bladder on ultrasound has a thin, hyperechoic smooth wall with anechoic fluid within. It is fixed at its caudal portion (trigone) to the cervix.

The ureters are hollow, muscular tubes not usually seen on ultrasound unless pathologically dilated.

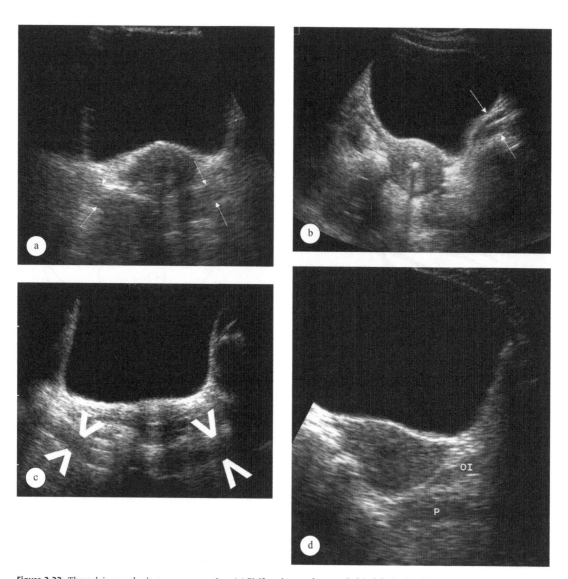

Figure 3.23 The pelvic muscles in transverse section. (a) Piriformis muscles seen behind the body of the uterus (arrows). (b) Iliopsoas (arrows) is demonstrated by angling slightly laterally. (c) Levator ani (arrowheads) at the level of the vagina. (d) The obturator internuis (OI) may be demonstrated lateral to the piriformis (P).

They are approximately 30 cm in length and pass anterior to the internal iliac artery and posterior to the ovary. Their relationship to the reproductive organs is important in cases of pelvic pathology, which may give rise to obstructive uropathy.

It is possible to identify the vesicoureteric junction in a transverse scan through the bladder base, and the ureteric jet may be clearly demonstrated using colour Doppler as it enters the bladder (Fig. 3.24).

Anatomical changes related to age

The uterus and ovaries vary in size according to age. Neonatal and paediatric appearances are discussed

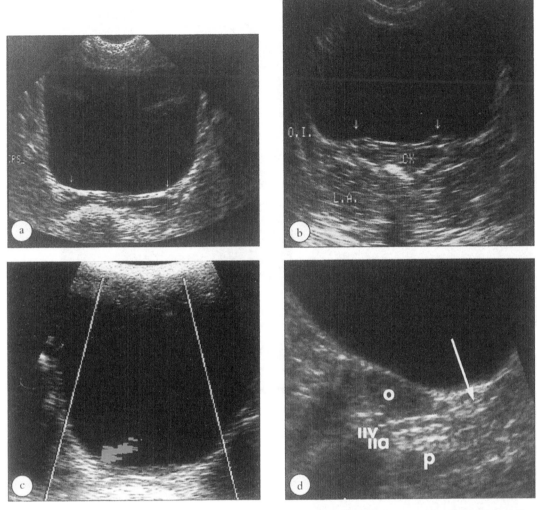

Figure 3.24 Ultrasonic appearances of the ureters. In transverse section, the ureters may be traced down as they travel medially, (a) and enter the bladder base (b). (c) At this level the ureteric jets may be demonstrated with colour Doppler. O.I., obturator internus; CX, cervix; L.A., levator ani. In longitudinal section, (d) the ureter may sometimes be seen as a tiny tube (arrow) between the ovary (o) and iliac vessels. iiv, internal iliac vein; iia, internal iliac artery; p, piriformis.

in Chapter 8 and postmenopausal pelvic organs in Chapter 4. A comparison of normal anatomical appearances with age is given in Table 3.1.

A simple formula for estimation of ovarian volume is:

$$\text{Volume (cm}^3) = \text{length} \times \text{width} \times \text{anteroposterior}$$
$$\text{diameter} \times 0.53$$

Later in life, at and following menopause, the uterus and ovaries atrophy. This regression in size is a gradual process and in the early postmenopausal phase the organs can appear ultrasonically very similar to those of the reproductive years. As in the premenarchal stage, the cervix is larger than the corpus. In the normal elderly patient, the endometrial echo, although thin, should still be demonstrated. The

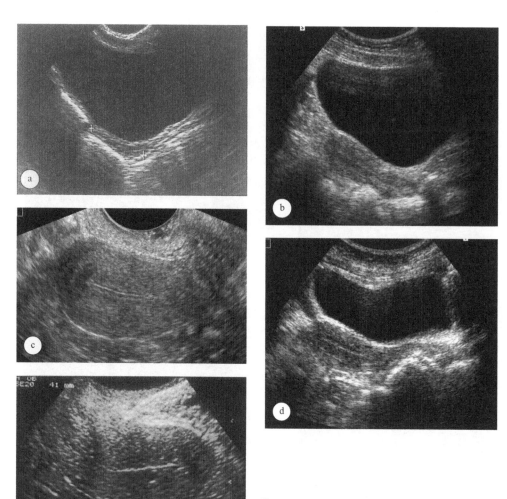

Figure 3.25 The differing appearances of the uterus with age.
(a) Paediatric (b and c); adult uterus transabdominal and transvaginal
scan; (d and e) postmenopausal uterus transabdominal and
transvaginal scan.

normal uterus at this stage is of uniform echogenicity but the ovaries become increasingly difficult to
image unless cysts are present (Fig. 3.25).

Physiology of reproduction

The female reproductive years occupy an average
35–40 years between puberty and menopause. The
standard hormonal cycle is 28 days, although it is
widely recognised that this is an arbitrary figure and
that there are variations to this pattern.

Throughout each normal cycle, the endometrium
and ovaries undergo changes brought about by
the hormones secreted by the pituitary gland –
follicle-stimulating hormone (FSH), luteinising hormone (LH) and prolactin. The ovaries themselves are

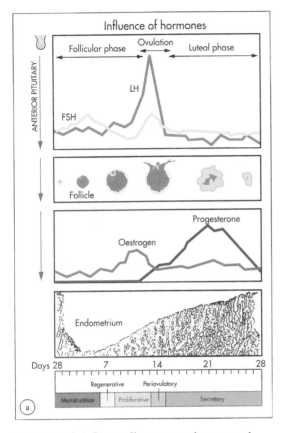

Figure 3.26 The influence of hormones on the uterus and ovaries. FSH, Follicle-stimulating hormone; LH, luteinising hormone.

also active and secrete oestrogen and progesterone (Fig. 3.26).

The purpose of these hormones is to produce a mature ovum for fertilisation, prepare the endometrium for the fertilised ovum and support the pregnancy in its early stages.

During the proliferative, or initial, phase of the cycle, FSH influences the immature follicles to develop, resulting in a dominant follicle being produced. Around day 14 of cycle, when the oestrogen levels are high, LH stimulates ovulation. During this period, the endometrium thickens and ripens. Following ovulation, during the secretory phase, the ovary secretes progesterone, FSH and oestrogen levels diminish and the follicular wall collapses forming the corpus luteum. If pregnancy does not occur, the endometrium becomes thickened and menstruation takes place on or around the 28th day.

Ultrasound appearances

Changes in the endometrium and ovaries can be well demonstrated sonographically using a high-frequency TV transducer (Figs. 3.27 and 3.28).

It is important to remember that the endometrium is a three-dimensional structure, and to scan it fully by angling the transducer from left to right uterine horn in longitudinal section, and from cervix to fundus in transverse section. In this way the operator

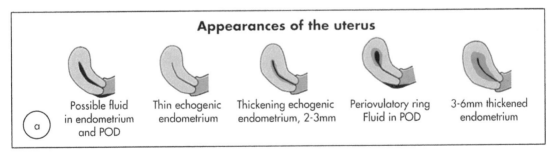

Figure 3.27 (a) The uterus in a normal cycle. POD, pouch of Douglas.

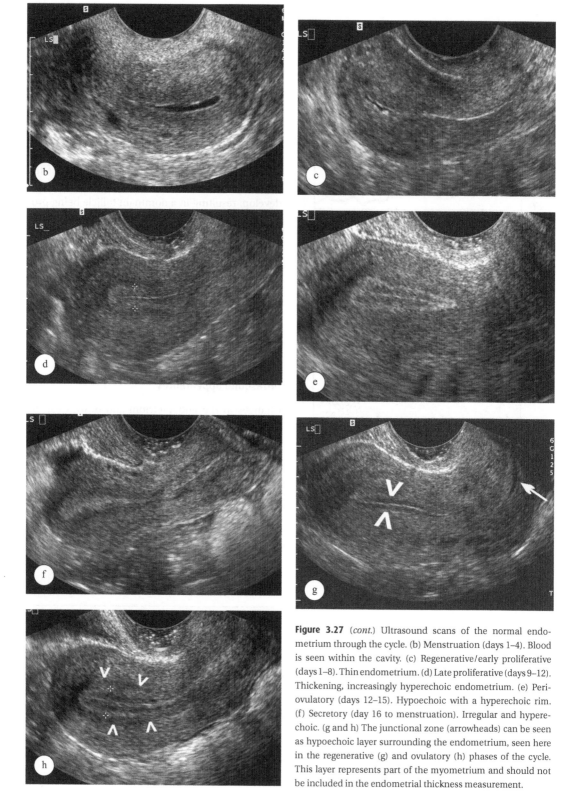

Figure 3.27 (*cont.*) Ultrasound scans of the normal endometrium through the cycle. (b) Menstruation (days 1–4). Blood is seen within the cavity. (c) Regenerative/early proliferative (days 1–8). Thin endometrium. (d) Late proliferative (days 9–12). Thickening, increasingly hyperechoic endometrium. (e) Periovulatory (days 12–15). Hypoechoic with a hyperechoic rim. (f) Secretory (day 16 to menstruation). Irregular and hyperechoic. (g and h) The junctional zone (arrowheads) can be seen as hypoechoic layer surrounding the endometrium, seen here in the regenerative (g) and ovulatory (h) phases of the cycle. This layer represents part of the myometrium and should not be included in the endometrial thickness measurement.

Appearances of the ovary

| Small follicles 1-2mm | Growth of dominant follicle | Cumulus oophorus | Ovulation | Corpus luteum | |

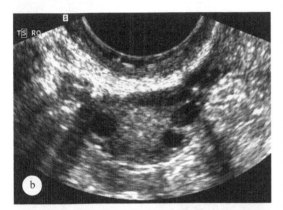
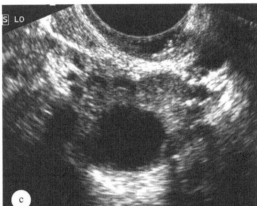
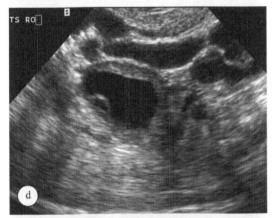
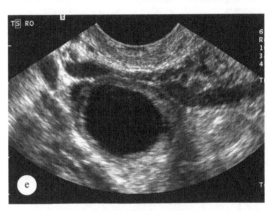
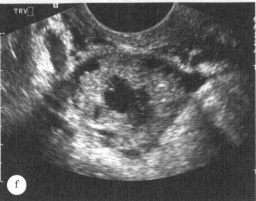

Figure 3.28 (a) The appearances of the dominant ovary. Ultrasound appearances of the dominant ovary through the cycle: (b) Regenerative (days 1–8): small follicles. (c) Proliferative (days 9–13): dominant follicle growing. (d) Ovulatory (days 13–14): cumulus oophorus seen in dominant follicle. (e) Early secretory (day 15 onwards). Corpus luteum. (f) Late secretory. Regression of corpus luteum.

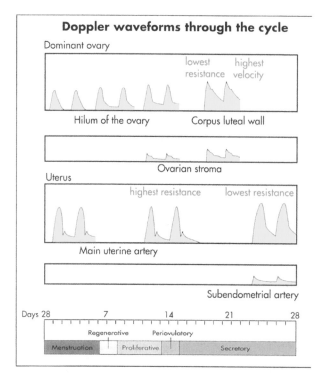

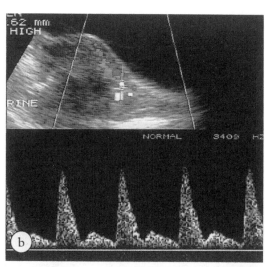

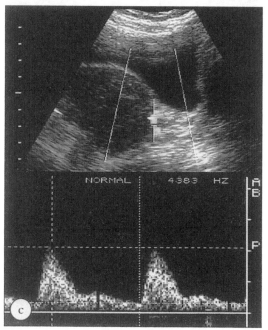

Figure 3.29 Doppler spectra of dominant ovarian and uterine waveforms through the cycle.

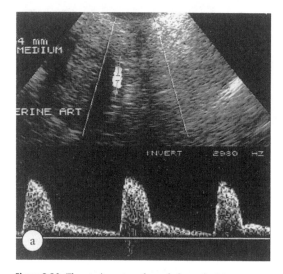

Figure 3.30 (*cont.*)

Figure 3.30 The uterine artery through the cycle. (a) Proliferative phase. (b) Postovulatory phase of highest resistance. (c) Mid to late secretory (or luteal) phase – lowest resistance

may identify focal abnormalities which may not be apparent on a midline longitudinal section.

Ultrasound appearances of the normal endometrium (Fig. 3.27)

During the early proliferative or regenerative stage, the endometrium appears as a thin reflective line in the uterine cavity.

At ovulation, the endometrium is hypoechoic, surrounded by a prominent, highly reflective echo, giving rise to the term 'triple-line' echo sign.[6]

Just before menstruation, the endometrium can be visualised as a thick hyperechoic structure passing centrally down the uterine cavity.

During menses, it is possible to visualise the endometrial cavity separated by low-level echoes representing blood and mucus.

Just below the endometrium it is often possible to see a hypoechoic, subendometrial 'halo' which represents the junctional zone between the endometrium and myometrium (Fig. 3.27g and 3.27h). This actually consists of normal myometrium[7] which comprises tightly packed mucosal cells with increased vascularity, and should not be included in the measurement of endometrial thickness.

Peristaltic waves within the endometrium have been identified on ultrasound, passing towards the cervix in menses, and towards the fundus in midcycle. These can best be appreciated by playing a video of the scan at a fast speed.[8]

The endometrium of a normal postmenopausal woman is thin (less than 4 mm) and hyperechoic,[9] mostly composed of the basalis layer. It is particularly important when scanning in cases of postmenopausal bleeding to identifiy the endometrial echo, and to examine it fully. Lack of a demonstrable endometrial echo is a highly suspicious finding and may indicate an invasive malignant process in a small number of cases.

Appearances of the ovary (Fig. 3.28)

During the regenerative and early proliferative stage the ovaries contain several immature follicles, typically less than 1 cm, within the ovarian tissue.

As the cycle progresses to ovulation, a dominant follicle measuring up to 2.0 cm can be seen. It is

possible to have more than one dominant follicle. In 60–65% of cases, the cumulus oophorus can be imaged between 12 and 24 hours prior to ovulation.[4] Ultrasonically, this appears as a small hyperechoic focus adherent to the follicular wall (Fig. 3.28d).

The collapsed walls of the dominant follicle are then apparent during the early secretory phase. Haemorrhagic changes also occur, demonstrated as low-level echoes within the collapsing corpus luteum, which also has a less defined outline. In some cases, fluid can also be seen in the pouch of Douglas.[6]

In postmenopausal women, the ovaries shrink and atrophy, often being more difficult to locate on ultrasound. With improvements in technology it is now common to see small cysts within the postmenopausal ovary and these are of no significance provided they are small (less than 5 cm) and simple (anechoic and smooth-walled).[10]

Haemodynamics of the uterus and ovaries and the use of Doppler ultrasound

The blood supply to the uterus and ovaries fluctuates throughout the normal cycle. These physiological changes can be appreciated using Doppler ultrasound (Fig. 3.29).

Both the ovary and endometrium exhibit angiogenesis – the formation of new blood vessels – during the course of the normal cycle. These 'new vessels' have low-resistance vasculature characterised by increased end-diastolic flow velocities with a low resistance index value. This phenomenon is also well recognised in pathological processes, such as the development of malignant tumours,[11] and the use of Doppler is therefore non-specific, particularly in premenopausal women.

Uterine arteries

The main uterine arteries, located just laterally to the region of the cervix, have a high resistance pattern with low end-diastolic flow and a notch (Fig. 3.30), and should not be confused with the iliac artery, which lies lateral to the uterine artery. The common and external iliac arteries exhibit

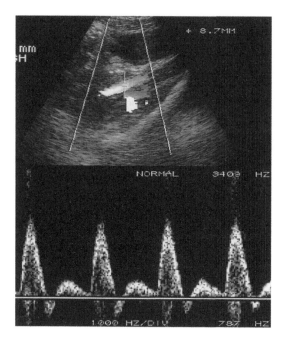

Figure 3.31 High-resistance, triphasic waveform from the iliac artery.

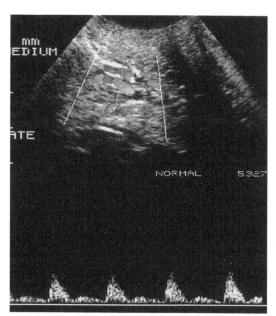

Figure 3.32 Low-velocity waveform from arcuate arteries within the myometrium.

very-high-resistance, triphasic flow with a reverse component; the internal iliac artery is less pulsatile but still exhibits a high-resistance, notched waveform with very little end-diastolic flow (Fig. 3.31).

Waveforms and resistance index measurements are more consistently reproducible from the main uterine artery than from its smaller, low-velocity, arcuate branches and the artery tends to be more easily visualised in premenopausal than postmenopausal patients. Vessels situated within the uterus, just below the endometrium, are more difficult to locate as they are of much lower velocity. The Doppler waveforms from these are therefore of low amplitude and tend to have a poorly defined envelope, making measurements prone to error (Fig. 3.32).

In a normal cycle, the resistance of the uterine artery is at its highest (lowest end-diastolic flow velocity) 1–2 days after ovulation – i.e. around cycle day 16.[12–14] It is at its lowest (having greatest end-diastolic velocity) during the mid to late luteal phase. Although it is more difficult to estimate velocity accurately in the tortuous pelvic vessels, an increase in velocity has also been noted during the same period. This is thought to correlate loosely with an increase in uterine perfusion, which would be logical at this time of possible implantation.

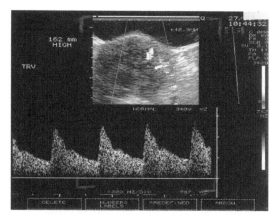

Figure 3.33 Decreased uterine artery resistance with fibroids.

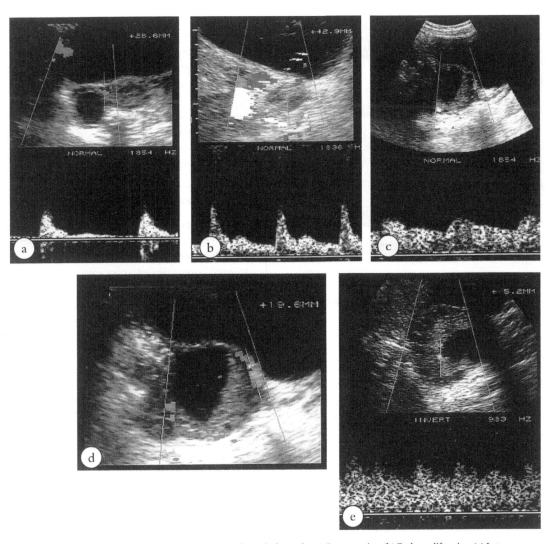

Figure 3.34 Decreasing resistance of the ovarian artery through the cycle. (a) Regenerative. (b) Early proliferative. (c) Late proliferative. (d) Periovulatory. (e) Secretory – wall of corpus luteum.

Although the uterine artery on the dominant side has been noted to have a slightly lower resistance index than the contralateral artery,[14] there is considerable overlap between the values, and the difference is small.

Several factors may be responsible for altering the resistance to flow of the uterine arteries, and these must be taken into account when interpreting Doppler information. A lower resistance index is seen in late luteal phase, in women on hormone replacement therapy, tamoxifen, and in the presence of uterine fibroids (Fig. 3.33). Malignancy such as endometrial carcinoma or uterine sarcoma is also associated with a lower uterine artery resistance index.

Uterine artery resistance increases with age, and a high resistance index may also be associated

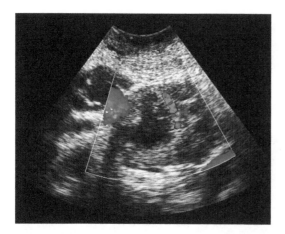

Figure 3.35 Typically increased vascularity around the wall of the corpus luteum.

with infertility, including tubal damage and endometriosis.

Ovarian arteries

As with the uterine arteries, but to an even greater degree, the resistance of the ovarian arteries is affected by cyclical, physiological changes, which are much greater in the dominant than the non-dominant ovary (Fig. 3.29). Downstream resistance is greatest (lowest end-diastolic flow) during days 1–8 of the cycle, with maximum resistance occurring around day 8.[14] (Days 1–8, therefore, make a good 'window' during which to examine the ovaries of pre-menopausal women, as low resistance is less likely at this time and misinterpretation of Doppler information is minimised.) Resistance to flow then gradually decreases from day 8 as the dominant follicle develops and ruptures around day 14. Resistance is at its lowest during the luteal phase, days 16–21, with the wall of the corpus luteum displaying the most intense colour pattern. It is at this time that the vessels are technically easiest to visualise. A gradual increase of resistance is then observed through to the regenerative phase (Fig. 3.34).[15,16]

These changes are most pronounced in the corpus luteum (Fig. 3.35).

The contralateral, non-dominant ovary tends to maintain a relatively high resistance throughout the cycle. In fact, it may be quite difficult to demonstrate any colour Doppler at all within the stroma, depending on the sensitivity of the ultrasound system used.

Identification of Doppler signals in the ovaries becomes increasingly difficult in the postmenopausal woman and usually demonstrates a low-velocity, high-resistance pattern.

Doppler ultrasound – key points

- Doppler information may be used to complement morphological information and should never be interpreted in isolation
- Normal Doppler waveforms vary with the stage of the menstrual cycle
- With less sensitive equipment, it may be difficult to visualise any Doppler flow in the ovary, particularly the non-dominant one
- Physiological and pathological Doppler waveforms can be indistinguishable
- False-positive Doppler results are therefore less common in postmenopausal women

---

REFERENCES

1. J. A. Rock and S. M. Markham, Developmental anomalies of the reproductive tract. In *Fertility: Evaluation and Treatment*, ed. W. R. Keye, R. J. Chang, R. W. Reber and M. R. Sules. (Philadelphia: W. B. Saunders, 1992).

2. M. Sanford, M. D. Markham and T. B. Waterhouse, Structural anomalies of the reproductive tract. *Current Opinion in Obstetrics and Gynecology* 4 (1992), 867–73.

3. A. Lev-Toaff, L. Pinheiro, G. Bega *et al.*, Three dimensional multiplanar sonohysterography. *Journal of Ultrasound in Medicine*, **20** (2001), 295–306.

4. I. E. Timor-Tritsch and S. Rottem (eds), *Transvaginal Sonography* (New York: Elsevier, 1988).

5. R. Warwick and P. Williams (eds), *Gray's Anatomy*, 35th edn. (Longman, 1973).

6. D. Gratton, C. Harrington, S. Holt and E. Lyons, Normal pelvic anatomy using transvaginal ultrasound. *Obstetrics and Gynecology Clinics of North America*, **18** (1991), 4.

7. R. Tetlow, I. Richmond, J. Greenman *et al.*, Histological ana-
    lysis of the uterine junctional zone as seen by transvaginal
    ultrasound. *Ultrasound in Obstetrics and Gynaecology*, **14**
    (1999), 188–93.

8. K. de Vries, E. A. Lyons, G. Ballard *et al.*, Contractions of the
    inner third of the myometrium. *American Journal of Obstet-
    rics and Gynecology*, **162** (1990), 679–82.

9. B. Gull, B. Karlsson, I Milsom *et al.*, Transvaginal sonogra-
    phy of the endometrium in a representative sample of post-
    menopausal women. *Ultrasound in Obstetrics and Gynae-
    cology*, **7** (1996) 322–7.

10. L. Valentin, L. Skoog and E. Epstein, Frequency and type
    of adnexal lesions in autopsy material from post-
    menopausal women: ultrasound study with histological
    correlation. *Ultrasound in Obstetrics and Gynecology*, **22**
    (2003), 284–9.

11. A. Kurjak, I. Zalud and Z. Alfirevic, Evaluation of adnexal
    masses with transvaginal color ultrasound. *Journal of Ultra-
    sound Medicine*, **10** (1991), 295–7.

12. P. Sladkevicius, L. Valentin and K. Marsal, Blood flow velo-
    city in the uterine and ovarian arteries during the normal
    menstrual cycle. *Ultrasound in Obstetrics and Gynecology*,
    3 (1993), 199.

13. R. K. Goswamy and P. C. Steptoe, Doppler ultrasound studies
    of the uterine artery in spontaneous ovarian cycles. *Human
    Reproduction*, **3** (1988), 721–6.

14. M. C. W. Scholtes, J. W. Wladimiroff, H. J. M. van Rijen and
    W. C. J. Hop, Uterine and ovarian flow velocity waveforms
    in the normal menstrual cycle: a transvaginal study. *Fertility
    and Sterility*, **52** (1989), 981–5.

15. L. T. Merce, D. Garces, M. J. Barco and F. de la Fuente, Intra-
    ovarian Doppler velocimetry in ovulatory, dysovulatory and
    anovulatory cycles. *Ultrasound in Obstetrics and Gynecol-
    ogy*, **2** (1992), 197.

16. K. Hata, T. Hata, D. Senoh *et al.*, Change in ovarian arterial
    compliance during the human menstrual cycle assessed by
    Doppler ultrasound. *British Journal of Obstetrics and Gynae-
    cology*, **97** (1990), 163–6.

4

Pathology of the uterus, cervix and vagina

Josephine M. McHugo

Birmingham Women's Hospital, Birmingham

Introduction

Ultrasound is the appropriate first investigation for the majority of pelvic symptoms in the female. It is however very operator-dependent and when used by appropriately trained personnel with appropriate equipment is cost-effective and safe. Transvaginal scanning is essential to increase the diagnostic accuracy of ultrasound and should be used in all cases unless there is a specific contraindication, such as in the paediatric population. It is essential that transabdominal ultrasound is also performed in order that the large fibroid uterus or other masses can be fully assessed in addition to imaging transvaginally.

There is a need for a meticulous approach to scanning in all cases so that significant pathology is not missed. The sonographer, having completed the ultrasound examination, must then issue an appropriate report. A structured report is also an essential part of the examination and should not only include the biographical details of the patient but also the salient ultrasound findings, both normal and abnormal, followed by either a definite diagnosis if this is possible, or a differential diagnosis.

Further investigations or definitive management can then be arranged.

The sonographer performing the examination should be clearly identified in the report.

A report that is structured in this way will allow retrospective audit of the ultrasound findings relative to operative findings and histology. This audit of accuracy of the ultrasound to histological outcome is essential for best practice.

In many situations the accuracy of transvaginal ultrasound is sufficient for further management of the patient but in some cases additional imaging such as magnetic resonance imaging (MRI) will be appropriate.

This chapter aims to outline the ultrasound findings of the common pathologies of the uterus, cervix and vagina.

The ultrasound findings must always be interpreted in the context of the clinical symptoms, age and hormonal status of the patient being scanned. It is therefore essential that each request for a pelvic ultrasound contains sufficient clinical information.

For clarity, this chapter with be divided into pathologies involving the myometrium, endometrium, cervix and vagina. For the ultrasound to be clinically useful the sonographer needs to have an understanding of the information that the referring clinician requires in order to manage the patient appropriately. The major decision is whether the ultrasound abnormality is responsible for the symptoms or is an incidental finding.

Similarly there is a need to assess the risk of malignancy. To this end there is a need to work in a multidisciplinary team, not only for appropriate management of the individual patient but also to audit outcome and effectiveness of ultrasound.

The uterus

Myometrium

Fibroids (leiomyomata)

Fibroids are benign tumours of the smooth muscle of the uterus and are the commonest gynaecological tumour, being present in up to 40% of women over 40 years. There is an increased incidence in women of Afro-Caribbean origin. Fibroids most commonly occur in the uterine body but are also found in the cervix or broad ligament. Histologically they are composed mainly of smooth muscle. The smooth-muscle fibres are arranged in dense concentric rings which are well demarcated from the surrounding normal myometrium, and it is this arrangement which is responsible for the ultrasound appearances.

These benign tumours are hormone-dependent, being associated with relatively high levels of oestrogen, and are frequently multiple. The incidence therefore increases with age until the menopause, and fibroids do not occur until well after the onset of puberty. Following the menopause the majority of fibroids reduce in size. Fibroids often enlarge in pregnancy and if they rapidly increase in size may outgrow their blood supply, resulting in central necrosis (red degeneration.) As with any ischaemic, necrotic process this results in considerable pain. Hormone replacement and tamoxifen can also stimulate growth. Fibroids, being oestrogen-dependent, respond to medical management and antioestrogen therapy with gonadotrophin-releasing hormone antagonist is of benefit to aid fibroid shrinkage.

Clinical symptoms

The clinical symptoms depend on the size and site of the fibroids. Fibroids that impinge into the endometrial cavity are defined as submucous. Submucous fibroids distort the uterine cavity and often result in menstrual problems, usually menorrhagia and dysmenorrhoea. Fibroids projecting from the outer uterine surface are termed subserosal, as they lie under the serosal surface of the uterus, and many of these

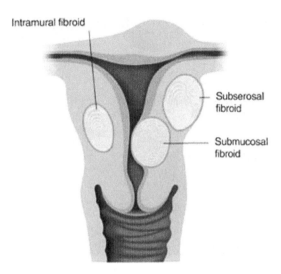

Figure 4.1 Diagram of fibroids.

remain asymptomatic. Fibroids within the myometrial mass that are neither subserosal nor submucous are termed intramural. Figure 4.1 outlines the possible sites of fibroids.

In some situations the fibroid may enlarge with a relatively thin stalk maintaining continuity to the myometrium. These are termed pedunculated. It is this continuity with the myometrium which is important to define with ultrasound, particularly if the fibroid projects into the broad ligament, as confusion with adenxal masses can occur if continuity with the myometrium is not identified. Submucosal pedunculated fibroids can prolapse into or through the cervical canal. These present clinically with pain, often dysmenorrhoea, but can also present with intermenstrual bleeding. Pedunculated fibroids, having a relatively narrow stalk, can undergo torsion which results in compromise of the vascular supply presenting with acute pain.

An enlarged fibroid uterus can result in pressure symptoms on the bladder or, if the uterus is retroverted, rectal symptoms. A markedly enlarged uterus presents as an abdominal mass and, rarely, can result in acute urinary retention. Following the menopause or after a period of rapid growth and degeneration, such as in pregnancy, fibroids often regress with the

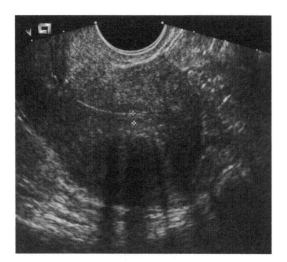

Figure 4.2 Posterior fibroid showing distal acoustic shadowing.

deposition of calcium. The calcium may be either punctate or circumferential.

Ultrasound appearances

Fibroids may be single or multiple, subserosal, intramural, submucous or pedunculated. These are very variable but are always well demarcated from the normal myometrium.

The dense nature of the abnormal smooth-muscle fibres results in loss of the normal homogeneous ultrasound appearances of the myometrium [Fig. 4.2) and acts as a stronger reflector than the normal myometrium. Therefore there is usually a degree of acoustic shadowing seen posterior to the fibroid.

This is more marked with a calcified fibroid, which is a stronger reflector (Fig. 4.3).

The reflectivity relative to the surrounding myometrium is variable; most is of lower reflectivity, but increased reflectivity is not an infrequent finding (Fig. 4.4).

Fibroids show a classical vascular supply with circumferential vessels, which are easily demonstrated using Doppler (Fig. 4.5).

The ultrasound report should describe the site, size and number of fibroids with particular reference to any distortion of the uterine cavity. It is vital

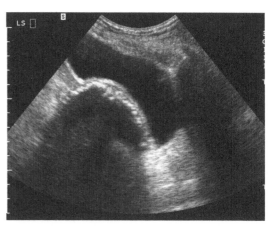

Figure 4.3 Transabdominal scan of a uterus with calcified fibroids, demonstrating strong acoustic shadowing.

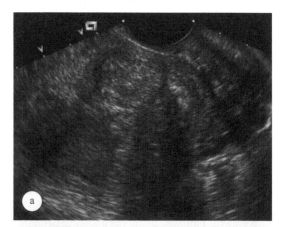

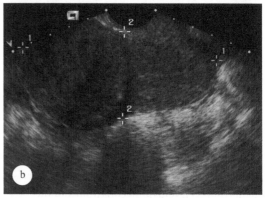

Figure 4.4 Sagittal image showing the varying reflectivity of fibroids: (a) a relative hyperechoic pattern and (b) a hypoechoic pattern of different fibroids.

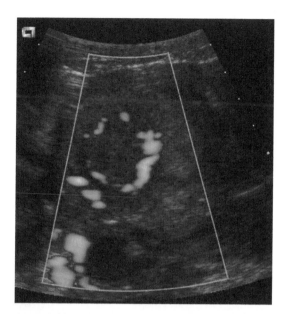

Figure 4.5 Power Doppler of a fibroid demonstrating circumferential vessels.

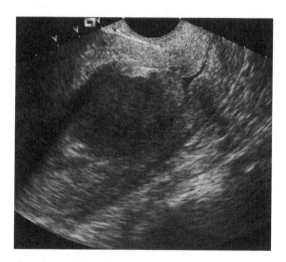

Figure 4.6 A submucosal fibroid.

to differentiate an endometrial polyp from a small fibroid, this being apparent by a combination of the acoustic pattern and the vascular supply (see endometrial disease, below) (Fig. 4.6).

In pregnancy the location and size of the fibroid relative to the cervical canal and the presenting fetal part are important. A relatively large fundal fibroid will not obstruct labour whereas smaller cervical fibroids may.[1]

A large fibroid uterus can cause a mass effect with partial obstruction of the distal ureters. Ultrasound examination of the upper renal tract and bladder voiding are therefore appropriate for a markedly enlarged fibroid uterus.

Degenerating fibroids create bizarre ultrasound appearances with central areas of necrosis showing as fluid-filled areas. In the acute phase these are very tender.

Diagnostic dilemmas

A pedunculated fibroid extending into the broad ligament may suggest a solid adnexal mass – careful examination should demonstrate the continuity with the myometrium.[2]

A retroverted normal uterus may suggest a fibroid on transabdominal scanning. This confusion is readily avoided by transvaginal scanning.

A bicornuate uterus may be confused with a fibroid but, by careful examination of the endometrial cavities, two separate uterine cavities and the overlying myometrium will be apparent. Examination in the later part of the menstrual cycle is particularly helpful in this circumstance as the endometrium will be more readily seen.

Small submucous fibroids may cause cornual obstruction and infertility secondary to tubal occlusion (Fig. 4.7).

Distortion of the endometrial cavity interferes with implantation and it is important to identify a normal cavity prior to embryo transfer in infertility programmes.

In pregnancy the non-gravid horn of a bicornuate uterus may appear as a fibroid if the endometrial cavity in this horn is not appreciated.

Larger fibroids will interfere with the normal enlargement of the pregnant uterus, resulting in second-trimester fetal loss, although this is relatively uncommon.[1] Fibroids can undergo rapid growth in pregnancy, outgrowing the blood supply, resulting in red degeneration causing acute pain.

A large fibroid low in the uterus can obstruct labour.

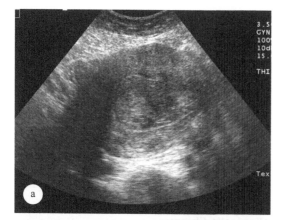

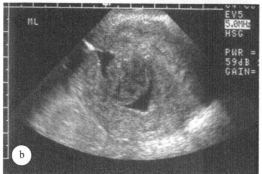

Figure 4.7 (a) An intracavitary submucosal fibroid, demonstrating some degeneration, with posterior acoustic enhancement, in a patient with infertility. (The differential diagnosis for these appearances would be of an endometrial polyp.) (b) A cornual fibroid.

A Braxton Hicks contraction in pregnancy may simulate a fibroid but if the uterus is scanned over a 20-min period the transient deformity caused by a contraction will disappear.

MRI of the uterus is extremely helpful and is essential if embolisation of the fibroids is being considered. T2 images define the zonal anatomy and readily identify the location of the fibroids in relation to the endometrial cavity (Fig. 4.8) (Table 4.1).

Leiomyosarcoma

Whether this represents a primary tumour or is malignant change in a previously benign fibroid remains an area of debate but in most cases it is thought to result from malignant change in a benign

Table 4.1 Differential diagnosis of fibroids

Small intrauterine fibroid	Adenomyoma
	Endometrial polyp – generally hyperechoic
Large/pedunculated fibroid	Solid ovarian mass
	Faeces-laden colon
	Large-bowel tumour
	Lymphoma, lymph nodes
	Pelvic kidney
	Other adnexal masses – especially ovarian fibroma

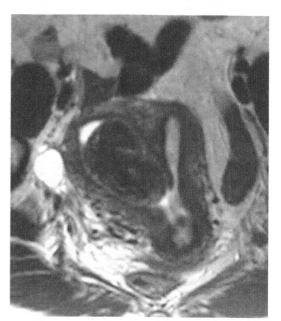

Figure 4.8 Magnetic resonance imaging of fibroids demonstrating their relationship to the endometrial cavity.

lesion. Its true incidence is unknown but it has a peak incidence at 50–60 years, being more common in Afro-Caribbeans and in those on tamoxifen.[3]

Sarcoma should be suspected when there is a solitary, solid, vascular mass in the myometrium which lacks the classical, well-demarcated borders of a fibroid and which shows loss of the circumferential blood vessels with central, turbulent flow within the tumour. There may be evidence of a rapid increase in size if the lesion has been scanned previously.

Ultrasound evidence of distant spread may be apparent.

The ultrasound features are non-specific and histological diagnosis is required whenever the suspicion of malignancy is raised.

Congenital abnormalities of the uterus

See Chapter 3. Fusion abnormalities should always be considered in the differential diagnosis of uterine abnormalities – many present around the time of puberty with obstructed features but some remain asymptomatic and result in confusing ultrasound appearances unless the sonographer is aware of this possibility.

Other uterine tumours

The following are all rare.

Mixed Müllerian carcinoma

Histologically this tumour is part carcinoma and part sarcoma, arising from pluripotential cells of the Müllerian duct system. There are rapidly invasive tumours with a poor prognosis and very variable ultrasound and MRI appearance.[4]

Uterine metastases

These are uncommon, but primary breast and stomach carcinomas may rarely spread to the uterus. Ovarian metastatic disease may be associated. Generally, simple or multiple endometrial masses of varying echogenicity are found. Abnormal uterine bleeding is the usual mode of presentation.[5]

Associated ultrasound features of malignant disease such as adenopathy should be noted.

Lymphoma

Lymphomatous infiltration of the uterus and cervix usually presents as part of a generalised lymphomatous disorder. Ultrasound will normally show a focal echo-poor uterine mass or infiltrate.[6] Other signs of lymphomatous involvement in the liver, spleen and lymph nodes will suggest the diagnosis.

Lipoma

A lipoma is a rare condition affecting mainly postmenopausal women with a characteristic, well-

defined, highly echogenic appearance. The MRI computed tomography (CT) appearance is also characteristic of a fatty tumour.[7]

Endometrial disease

It is essential to recognise the appearances of the normal adult (see Chapter 3) and paediatric (see Chapter 8) in order to understand the spectrum of changes seen in pathology.

An appreciation of the normal appearances of the endometrium with respect to the age and hormonal status of the patient is also essential for an understanding of abnormal features seen on ultrasound. What may be entirely normal in the fertile patient who has regular cycles will be pathological in the pre-or postmenopausal patient.

Endometrial disease usually presents with menstrual disorders: intermenstrual bleeding in the fertile female and per vaginam bleeding in the postmenopausal patient. Cervical causes of bleeding should always be excluded with this symptomatology. Direct visual examination and cervical cytology are mandatory in all cases with menstrual disorders. Bleeding from other areas of the genital tract, e.g. the vulva, should be excluded and bleeding from the bladder and rectum should also be excluded. This is particularly true in paediatric and elderly patients where the exact site of the bleeding may be uncertain from the clinical history.

The aetiologies of abnormal vaginal bleeding are varied (Table 4.2).

It is essential to have sufficient clinical information in each patient and this must include the hormonal status and stage of the menstrual cycle as well as the presenting clinical symptoms. Fortunately, in most cases it is possible to elicit this from the patient by direct questioning if it is not provided by the referring physician.

Endometrial thickness

The endometrium, regardless of the stage in the menstrual cycle, should be of regular thickness and have a regular contour with a sharp, well-defined border between the endometrium and myometrium. In the normal postmenopausal patient a low reflective region between the endometrium and the

Table 4.2 Aetiology of abnormal vaginal bleeding

Uterus	Fibroids
	Adenomyosis
	Endometrial pathology
	Hyperplasia
	Polyp
	Carcinoma
	Pelvic inflammatory disease (PID)
	Chronic endometritis
	Oestrogen-producing ovarian tumour
	Postmenopausal atrophic endometritis
Cervix	Chronic cervicitis
	Polyp
	Carcinoma
Vagina	Atrophic vaginitis
	Infection
	Foreign body (retained tampon, pessary)
	Trauma
	Carcinoma
Vulva	Squamous carcinoma
	Melanoma
Other	Haematuria or rectal bleeding (mistaken for vaginal bleeding)
	Bleeding disorders
	Medications – heparin, warfarin

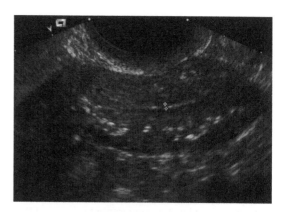

Figure 4.9 Sagittal scan showing the hypoechoic area between the thin, regular line of the endometrium and the homogeneous echo pattern of the myometrium. Note the calcification in the arcuate vessels of the uterus – a normal finding in the postmenopausal female.

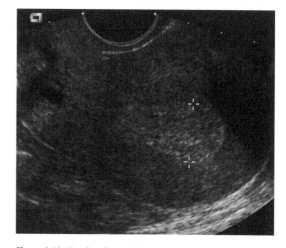

Figure 4.10 Focal endometrial thickening due to a polyp.

myometrium is apparent (Fig. 4.9). This regularity and boundary are of particular importance. The endometrial echo texture changes during the menstrual cycle but the texture should be uniform throughout the length of the endometrium. The measurement of the endometrial thickness is the maximum double thickness measured on a sagittal scan. It is vital to relate this measurement to the remainder of the endometrial thickness as minor increases can indicate significant pathology (Fig. 4.10). This is particularly true in the postmenopausal patient. Focal increases in thickness usually indicate polyps and interrogating the vascular supply with colour Doppler is useful as polyps will have a focal feeding vessel at the base (Fig. 4.11).

In the postmenopausal patient, an endometrial thickness greater than 4 mm is considered abnormal.[8–10]

In the menstrual years a thickness of up to 14 mm is considered normal (Table 4.3).

Abnormal focal thickening of the endometrium or focal abnormalities suggesting a submucous fibroid can be further investigated by the instillation of normal saline via a transcervical catheter (saline infusion sonohysterogram)[11] (Fig. 4.12). In this technique a soft catheter is placed under direct vision into the uterine cavity via the cervix. Once in position, normal saline is instilled into the uterine cavity at the same time as a transvaginal scan is being performed (Fig. 4.13). The fluid in the cavity accurately

Table 4.3 Endometrial thickness

Thin	Premenarche
	Cyclical change during menstrual cycle
	Oligomenorrhoea/amenorrhoea
	Oral contraceptive pill
	Post transcervical endometrial resection
Thick	Cyclical change during menstrual cycle
	Endometrial hyperplasia
	Endometrial polyp
	Endometrial carcinoma
	Medications hormone replacement therapy, tamoxifen
	Dysfunctional uterine bleeding
Apparent or pseudo-thickness	Retained products of conception
	Trophoblastic disease
	Haemato/pyometra

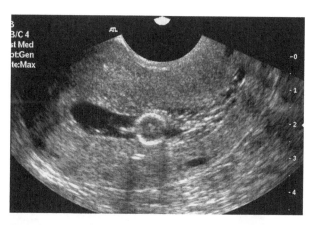

Figure 4.12 Saline infusion hysterosonography, demonstrating the balloon catheter within the lower part of the uterus and saline outlining the endometrial cavity.

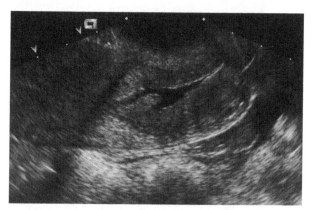

Figure 4.13 Saline within the uterine cavity outlines a small posterior endometrial polyp.

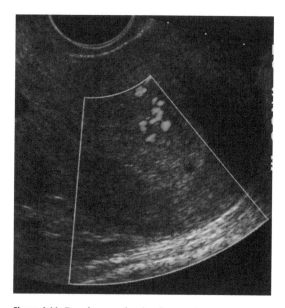

Figure 4.11 Doppler scan showing the vascular supply to an endometrial polyp.

demonstrates the endometrium.[12,13] This technique is increasingly employed by clinicians, but for many the advent of outpatient hysteroscopy is a procedure that is not only diagnostic but also allows biopsy and hysteroscopic polypectomy and is therefore considered more appropriate.[14] However saline hysterosonography is an appropriate option for monitoring tamoxifen if MRI is not employed.

Endometrial polyp

This is a common disorder, being found in 10% of women, and is defined as overgrowths of the endometrial glands, stroma and blood vessels that project into the cavity (Figs. 4.13 and 4.14).

They are frequently multiple on histology. The ultrasound appearances are of focal endometrial thickening, often with some cystic changes of the endometrium with feeding vessels seen at the

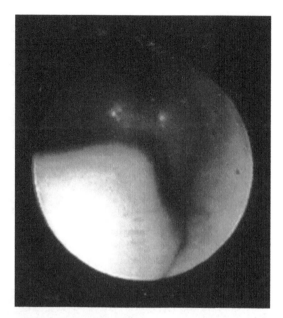

Figure 4.14 Hysteroscopy of a polyp.

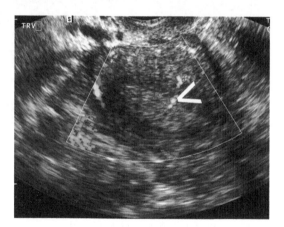

Figure 4.15 Ultrasound of a polyp with a feeding vessel (arrowhead) on power Doppler.

base (Fig. 4.15). The echogenicity is similar to the endometrium, which should distinguish these polyps from submucosal fibroids, in which the echogenicity is usually reduced.

Pedunculated endometrial polyps may protrude into the cervical canal.

Ultrasound appearances.   Polyps may be single or multiple, and are frequently small – usually < 1 cm. They tend to be hyperechoic, sometimes containing small cystic spaces. A feeding vessel can often be demonstrated from the base using colour or power Doppler.

Investigation of postmenopausal bleeding
This is a common symptom, resulting in 5% of gynaecological referrals.[10]

The aetiology of these symptoms is mainly from an atrophic endometrium in which the superficial blood vessels are friable and unsupported by the surrounding connective tissue, resulting in bleeding. In this case the endometrium is thin on ultrasound. Other causes of postmenopausal bleeding result in endometrial thickening and for the majority this is benign disease, but in 10% of symptomatic postmenopausal women endometrial carcinoma is present.

The measurement of endometrial thickness on ultrasound, using > 4 mm as the cut-off for abnormal, has an excellent negative predictive value in excluding endometrial pathology. However it has a poor positive predictive value for endometrial carcinoma or hyperplasia, therefore transvaginal ultrasound is employed as a first-line screening tool in the investigation of postmenopausal bleeding to exclude significant endometrial pathology. A positive ultrasound, when the endometrium is > 4 mm, requires further diagnostic investigation. Further demonstration of the endometrial–myometrial border, and irregularity of the endometrium, allows the detection of significant pathology when the thickness is ≤ 4 mm.

When the postmenopausal endometrium is atrophic, the ultrasound findings are of a thin endometrial stripe (Fig. 4.16).

Endometrial hyperplasia
Histologically four types of hyperplasia are seen in postmenopausal women:
1. metaplasia (usually squamous)
2. simple cystic hyperplasia
3. complex (adenomatous) hyperplasia
4. complex hyperplasia with atypia

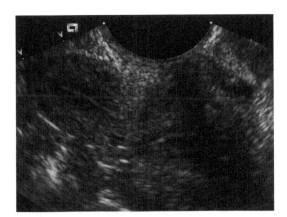

Figure 4.16 Scan showing thin and regular atrophic endometrium in a postmenopausal woman.

Table 4.4 International Federation of Gynecology and Obstetrics (FIGO) classification of endometrial cancer staging

Stage I	Carcinoma confined to the corpus
IA	The length of the uterine cavity is 8 cm or less
IB	The length of the uterine cavity is greater than 8 cm
Stage II	Carcinoma has involved corpus and cervix but has not extended outside the uterus
Stage III	Carcinoma has extended outside the uterus but not outside the true pelvis
Stage IV	Carcinoma has extended outside the true pelvis or has obviously involved the mucosa of the bladder or rectum
IVA	Carcinoma has spread to adjacent organs
IVB	Carcinoma has spread to distant organs

This normally results from excessive oestrogen stimulation (both endogenous and exogenous) and with unopposed progesterone there is an increased risk of endometrial cancer.[15] Tamoxifen, being weakly oestrogenic in postmenopausal women, increases the risk by two to six times.[16] Additional risk factors for endometrial carcinoma are obesity, diabetes and nulliparity.

The preinvasive nature of endometrial cancer is well established. The malignant potential of simple hyperplasia is 1–3% over 15 years, that of complex hyperplasia is 3–4%, and that of atypical hyperplasia is 23%.[17]

Endometrial carcinoma

This is the commonest gynaecological malignancy, with a peak incidence between 60 and 70 years. It is rarely seen before the menopause: only 3% of patients present under 40 years. The classification is based on the histological cell type – most are adenocarcimomas.

The tumour is manifest early in the disease process by symptoms of postmenopausal bleeding and is present in 10% of patients with this symptom.

It is essential in patients with per vaginam blood loss to exclude other causes of bleeding. Direct visual inspection of the cervix and cervical cytology is mandatory. Vulval causes of bleeding, e.g. squamous

carcinoma or melanoma, need to be considered, as do other non-genital bleeding sites, particularly the bladder or rectum. This is particularly true in the elderly when the origin of the bleeding is less certain from the clinical history.

Ultrasound findings Endometrial carcinoma has a thickened endometrium. The endometrial–myometrial border is irregular and there is loss of homogenicity of the endometrium.

Asymmetry of the myometrial thickness (indicating myometrial invasion) can also be demonstrated.

Disordered, turbulent intratumoral blood flow can be seen on colour or power Doppler (Fig. 4.17a and b).

As the disease is clinically apparent early in the disease process, spread to the broad ligament and lateral pelvic wall is rarely seen at presentation.

Staging, and hence prognosis and treatment, depends on myometrial invasion. Although this can be inferred by the depth of the myometrium seen on ultrasound, this is less accurate than MRI, which is the investigation of choice for staging (Fig. 4.18).

Endometrial cancer staging The tumour is staged clinically using the International Federation of Gynecology and Obstetrics (FIGO) classification (Table 4.4).

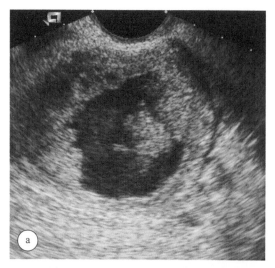

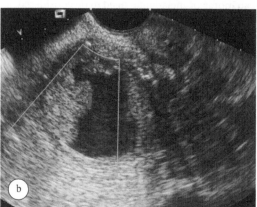

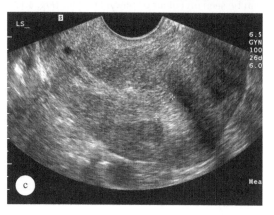

Figure 4.17

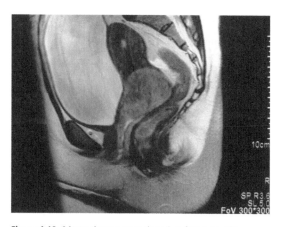

Figure 4.18 Magnetic resonance imaging demonstrating carcinoma of the cervix.

Medication

Oral contraceptive pill Generally, oestrogen and progesterone are combined and administered in a cyclical fashion. The endometrium may be expected to be thin and varies little during the menstrual cycle. Occasionally, slight uterine enlargement may be noted and multiple small randomly arranged cysts may be seen in the ovaries.

Hormone replacement therapy (HRT) HRT is commonly used for the treatment of menopausal symptoms and is also used in the treatment of premature ovarian failure. Many preparations are available but most combine oestrogen and progesterone and are given in a cyclical, sequential manner. Consequently cyclical changes in endometrial thickness are observed ultrasonographically with a thickness of up to 15 mm in the oestrogen phase, and the endometrium being relatively

Figure 4.17 (*cont.*) (a) Abnormal, thickened and irregular endometrium with echogenic fluid from carcinoma of the endometrium. (b) Vascular supply to the solid areas in carcinoma of the uterus. (c) Early endometrial carcinoma demonstrating an irregularly thickened endometrium with indistinct margins on ultrasound.

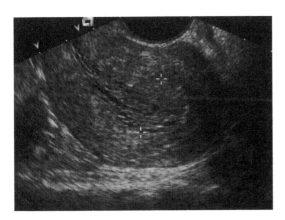

Figure 4.19 Sagittal scan of the uterus showing typical features of the endometrium, which is thickened with some cystic changes, in a patient taking tamoxifen.

less thick in the progesterone phase. Ultrasound assessment of endometrial thickness is best performed immediately after the progesterone phase of the cycle when the endometrium is likely to be thinnest. The majority of patients are scanned for unscheduled bleeding on HRT. The most important ultrasound sign in this group to suggest endometrial pathology is irregularity of the endometrium with abnormal vascularity.

Tamoxifen Tamoxifen is an oral synthetic antioestrogen compound with mild oestrogenic effects on the uterine properties. It is used as an adjuvant chemotherapeutic agent in the treatment of breast cancer. Tamoxifen, due to the oestrogenic effects, causes endometrial metaplasia, hyperplasia and carcinoma.[18] In patients receiving tamoxifen therapy, the normal risk of developing endometrial carcinoma is increased sixfold, with both pre- and postmenopausal women being affected.[19] Fifty per cent of women taking tamoxifen will develop some type of endometrial pathology after 6–36 months of treatment.[20]

Tamoxifen has characteristic ultrasound appearances of endometrial thickening with multiple abnormal small cystic spaces within the abnormal endometrium (Fig. 4.19). In addition it causes subendometrial cysts which can be indistinguishable from the endometrium on ultrasound. Therefore the true endometrial thickness is overestimated by ultrasound.

Ultrasound is therefore unreliable in the prediction of endometrial pathology in symptomatic women on tamoxifen. These women require histological correlation, which is best performed under direct hysteroscopic vision. Saline hysterosonography[21] (Fig. 4.20) is helpful in monitoring the endometrial irregularity more accurately but MRI is best as it differentiates the endometrium from the subendometrial cysts.

Ultrasound appearances The endometrium is thickened – almost always >10 mm. In addition it may be hyperechoic, irregular in outline, with cystic areas (<5 mm) and there may be polyps.

Gestational trophoblastic disease
This results from abnormal trophoblastic tissue and is therefore always associated with the products of conception, usually presenting with symptoms of pregnancy and no discernible fetus.

Three entities are recognised:
1. molar pregnancy
2. invasive mole
3. chorion carcinoma

These subdivisions can be considered as types with increasing invasive propensities: choriocarcinoma is the most invasive, with early lung metastases.[22]

In the majority the genetic make up of the tissue is of paternal origin. The abnormal trophoblastic tissue secretes high levels of beta-human choriono-gonadotrophic (βHCG) hormone, resulting in symptoms of nausea and vomiting. The abnormal tissue is prone to bleeding and per vaginam blood loss is a common symptom.

Ultrasound features of all types are of an endometrial mass with cystic spaces (Fig. 4.21). The high βHCG levels are associated with thecal luteal cysts of the ovaries.[23]

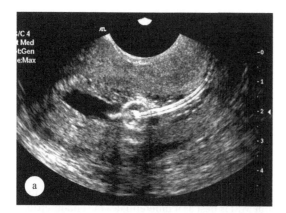

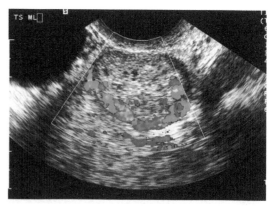

Figure 4.21 An area of trophoblastic invasion in the lower uterus, with peripheral vascularity demonstrated on colour Doppler.

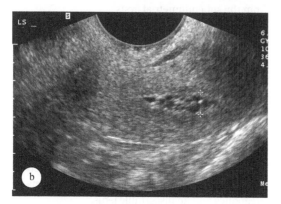

Choriocarcinoma Choriocarcinoma is treated by curettage and methotrexate therapy. Response and recurrence are monitored with serum βHCG levels, which allow excellent assessment of the response, of the disease to treatment. MRI and CT are useful to check for distant spread, most particularly to the lungs. Chemotherapy produces an excellent response, with a 90% cure rate.

Inflammatory conditions
Acute endometritis This condition is most commonly seen in the postpartum uterus, usually associated with retained products of conception which act as the foci for the infection. Similarly, postuterine instrumentation, including suction termination of pregnancy, is a significant risk factor.

The ultrasound appearances are of an enlarged tender uterus showing loss of the endometrial myometrial borders and echogenic retained products if present. There is a diffuse increase in the vascularity of the uterus due to the acute infection. If extensive, there will be additional signs of pelvic infections such as free or loculated fluid and the ultrasound signs of a tubo-ovarian abscess. The patient will be acutely unwell with fever and an elevated white cell count.[24]

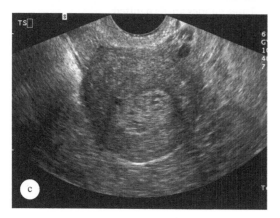

Figure 4.20 (a) Saline infusion hysterosonography of a tamoxifen endometrium, showing subendometrial cystic hyperplasia. (b) Cystic change on ultrasound in the endometrium of a patient on tamoxifen. (c) A polyp in a patient on tamoxifen, demonstrating cystic change.

Postoperative conditions

It is essential to have an understanding of the type of gynaecological surgery performed in order to understand the normal and abnormal postoperative features seen with ultrasound. It is normal to have a small collection of blood at the vault of the vagina immediately postoperatively following a hysterectomy and in a subtotal hysterectomy the cervix is left in situ. Abnormal postoperative collections are usually haematomas but these may become infected.

Ultrasound signs of infection include septation, echogenic fluid and increasing tenderness. In this situation ultrasound guided per vaginam drainage may be appropriate.

Post-caesarean section Following a lower-segment caesarean section, the uterus will usually appear entirely normal after 6 weeks. But in some patients, a small anterior deformity will be seen at the junction of the middle and lower uterine segments at the site of the surgical incision. This may have the ultrasound appearance of a small fibroid but its site and the clinical history should suggest the diagnosis. This minor abnormality is clinically insignificant (Fig. 4.22).

Adenomyosis Adenomyosis, in which ectopic endometrium 'invades' the myometrium, may be considered a variant of endometriosis. The two conditions are known to coexist in 20% of affected patients. Histologically, ectopic endometrial glands and stroma are found in the myometrium. The typical patient will be a multiparous woman in her 40s presenting with menorrhagia and dysmenorrhoea. This presentation contrasts with that of endometriosis whereby a nulliparous, infertile woman in her 20s or 30s is most likely to be affected. Adenomyosis may be associated with previous dilatation and curettage (D&C), caesarean section or elevated oestrogen levels. The disease is usually generalised but occasionally a localised focus, termed an adenomyoma, may be found.[25]

Ultrasound appearances The ultrasound appearances are variable and non-specific but usually there

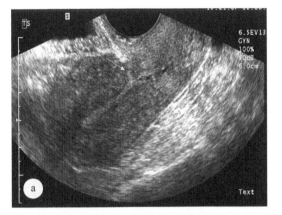

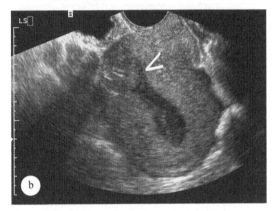

Figure 4.22 (a) Post-caesarean-section scar on ultrasound (arrow). (b) This lower-segment caesarean-section scar fills with fluid during a saline infusion hysterosonogram.

is slight enlargement of the uterus with loss of the homogenicity of the myometrium, without specific features of discrete fibroids. Occasionally tiny cystic areas within the myometrium can be discerned on transvaginal ultrasound, and hyperechoic areas, probably corresponding to areas of cyclic haemorrhage, have also been reported.

MRI is more specific and is the diagnostic imaging modality of choice (Fig. 4.23).

Asherman's syndrome

Intrauterine synechiae, or adhesions, result from overenthusiastic endometrial curettage during or

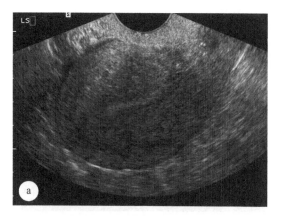

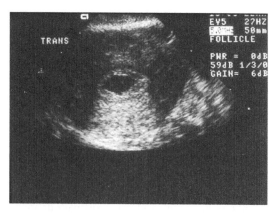

Figure 4.24 Asherman's syndrome demonstrating synechiae on saline infusion.

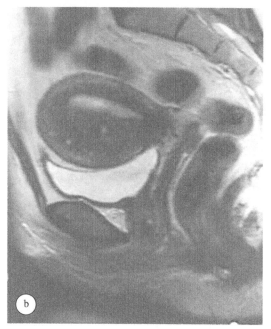

Figure 4.23 (a) The ultrasound features of adenomyosis may be subtle. This uterus is enlarged, with a heterogeneous myometrial texture and a slightly irregular endometrium. (b) Magnetic resonance imaging demonstrating adenomyosis.

following pregnancy. During the pregnancy the endometrium is more friable than normal and this may allow the complete removal of focal areas of endometrium. As a result, single or multiple bands of fibrous tissue completely or partially traverse the endometrial cavity. Similar adhesions may develop

post-myomectomy or post-caesarean section and in association with infection, i.e. endometritis, tuberculosis and schistosomiasis.

These adhesions may be an incidental finding at ultrasound but the patient may present with a history of dysmenorrhoea, oligomenorrhoea, infertility or recurrent miscarriage.

On ultrasound, the adhesions are usually seen as very small echogenic foci related to the endometrial cavity.[26] If there is fluid in the cavity, the adhesions may be better and more conclusively demonstrated. It is best diagnosed following saline infusion (Fig. 4.24).

Generally the diagnosis will be confirmed at hysterosalpingography or hysteroscopy, at which time the adhesions may be divided.

Intrauterine contraceptive device (IUCD)
These are a common form of contraception. Transvaginal ultrasound is the investigation of choice to locate the device. It should be situated high in the uterine cavity and placement outside of this should be considered abnormal and more likely to be ineffective. It is important to be aware of the differing ultrasound appearances of the various types of devices. This is particularly true of the Mirena coil, a device impregnated with levonorgestrel which is widely used for the symptomatic treatment of menorrhagia as well as for contraception. With the

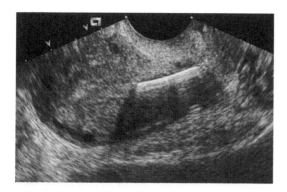

Figure 4.25 An intrauterine contraceptive device in the endometrial cavity.

Mirena the long arm is more echogenic than the T arm and for the unwary the ultrasound appearances suggest a coil that is abnormally low in the cavity.

Ultrasound appearances of IUCD The IUCD is usually a strong reflector with posterior acoustic shadowing (Fig. 4.25), lying within and along the endometrial cavity.

Abnormal positions There is approximately a 1:2000 risk of perforation of the device, usually into the myometrium, at insertion. In this situation the IUCD may be shown to lie outside the uterine cavity, i.e separate to the endometrium, rather than within it (Fig. 4.26).

Coils outside the uterus are rarely seen with ultrasound and any investigation where the coil cannot be identified with ultrasound merit an abdominal X-ray.

It is important to remember that even with the IUCD correctly sited pregnancy can occur and in this situation there is also an increased risk of an ectopic pregnancy.

The cervix

Investigation of cervical pathologies is by direct vision and cytology, although transvaginal scanning in the pregnant and non-pregnant female will

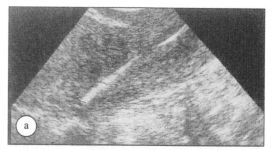

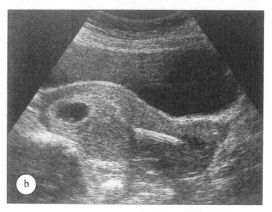

Figure 4.26 (a) Sagittal transvaginal scan showing an intrauterine contraceptive device (IUCD) penetrating the myometrium. (b) Sagittal transabdominal scan showing a 7-week gestation sac with an IUCD located in the cervix.

demonstrate the cervix if this area is carefully examined. However MRI with its excellent tissue characterisation is the imaging modality of choice.

Benign conditions
Nabothian cysts
These are epithelial inclusion cysts which develop in the endocervical canal, and are most commonly found in the perimenopausal period. These cysts develop as a result of chronic cervicitis which causes obstruction of the endocervical glands, resulting in retention of secretions. Nabothian cysts are asymptomatic and clinically insignificant.

Ultrasound appearances Nabothian cysts generally occupy a central position relating to cervical canal. They may be single or multiple (Fig. 4.27) and

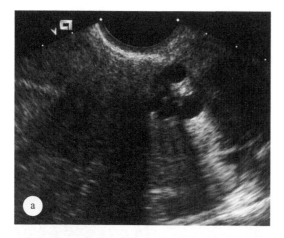

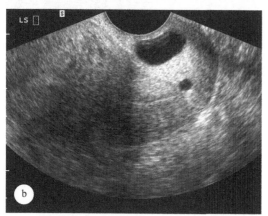

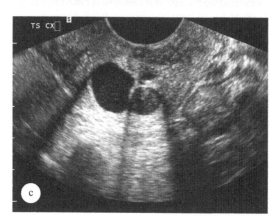

Figure 4.27 (a and b) Multiple nabothian cysts in the cervix. (c) One of these nabothian cysts contains echoes and debris.

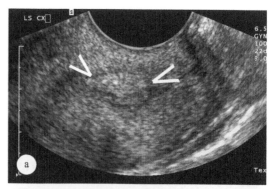

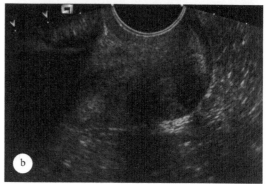

Figure 4.28 (a) A cervical fibroid (arrowsheads). The differential diagnosis on these appearances would be of a cervical polyp. (b) Cervical fibroid in a pregnant patient may potentially obstruct labour.

the size varies from a few millimetres to several centimetres, but they are generally < 1 cm.

They are usually echo-free, but some will contain confluent internal echoes.

Cervical fibroid

Cervical fibroids are uncommon, accounting for 8% of fibroids, the majority being in the uterine body. Most are small and asymptomatic with the same ultrasound features as the uterine fibroids described earlier in this chapter. However, when large cervical fibroids may be symptomatic due to their mass effect by producing either bladder compression with urinary frequency or in the pregnant patient by causing obstruction to labour (Fig. 4.28). MRI may be of value in clearly defining the position and size of the

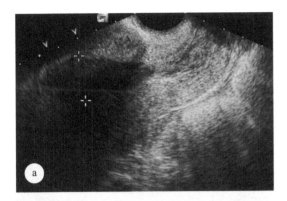

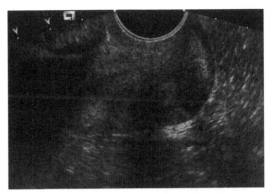

Figure 4.30 Echogenic small posterior cervical fibroid.

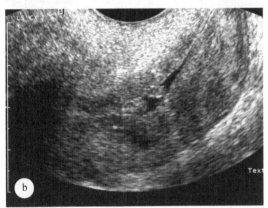

Figure 4.29 (a) Cervical polyp: hypoechoic area seen in the upper cervical canal. (b) Small endocervical polyps surrounded by a tiny amount of fluid in the cervix.

fibroid, particularly in late pregnancy, where ultrasound may not provide adequate visualisation of a cervical mass.

Cervical polyp

Clinically, cervical polyps are asymptomatic or present with intermenstrual bleeding and/or dysmenorrhoea. These polyps are benign and develop from hyperplastic cervical epithelium which results from chronic cervicitis. The polyps are generally small, measuring less than 1 cm, and appear echogenic ultrasonographically (Fig. 4.29). They may be pedunculated and occasionally may prolapse into the vagina where they may be mistaken for pedunculated endometrial polyps, or pedunculated submucosal fibroids (Fig. 4.30). Occasionally, colour flow Doppler may demonstrate a vascular pedicle.

Congenital cystic remnants of mesonephric origin are rarely seen.

Cervical carcinoma

Cervical carcinoma is the second most common malignancy in the UK, with 4000 new cases per year. This disease is often associated with multiple sexual partners from an early age and, as such, is increasing in frequency. Both cervical carcinoma and the preinvasive forms are associated with the human papillomavirus and herpes simplex type 2 virus. The average age of diagnosis is 45 years but increasingly younger women are involved. Histologically, 90% are squamous cell carcinomas arising from the ectocervix, with 10% being endocervical adenocarcinomata. Other forms of tumour are very rare.

The diagnosis is generally made clinically and histologically with many patients being identified by the National Screening Programme. Carcinoma-in-situ is a precancerous condition. Patients with advanced disease present with abnormal uterine bleeding, whether intermenstrual or postmenopausal, and/or with a vaginal discharge.

The tumour spreads via the lymphatics to the parametra and to local pelvic lymph nodes. Subsequently, these will spread to the iliac and para-aortic lymph nodes. The tumour metastasises haematologically to the liver and lungs but this is a late

Table 4.5 FIGO staging of cervical carcinoma

Stage 0	Carcinoma-in-situ
Stage I	Carcinoma confined to cervix
IA	Microinvasive (only diagnosed histologically)
IB	Clinically invasive carcinoma confined to cervix
Stage II	Carcinoma extends beyond the cervix but has not extended to the pelvic side wall. The carcinoma involves the vagina but not the lower third
IIA	No obvious parametrial involvement
IIB	Obvious parametrial involvement
Stage III	Carcinoma has extended to the pelvic side wall and/or the lower third of the vagina
IIIA	Lower third of the vagina involved
IIIB	Extension to pelvic side wall and/or hydronephrosis
Stage IV	Carcinoma has extended beyond the true pelvis and/or has clinically involved the bladder or rectum
IVA	Biopsy proves bladder or rectal tumour
IVB	Distant metastases beyond the pelvis

occurrence. Due to the close proximity of the tumour to the ureters, entrapment and invasion are common. This leads to hydroureter and hydronephrosis and renal impairment if bilateral. Nephrostomy or urinary stenting may be required in order to prevent renal failure.

Although transvaginal and transrectal ultrasound has some value in the staging of cervical carcinoma,[27] MRI must be regarded as the gold standard. Clinical staging and MRI may be combined in the management of the disease. The well-accepted FIGO staging is detailed in Table 4.5.

Generally, stage I and IIA tumours will be treated surgically with or without adjuvant radiotherapy. Stage IIB and above tumours are generally treated with radiotherapy whether external, intracavitary or both.

Ultrasound appearances Early tumours are not ultrasonographically identifiable. Slightly more advanced tumours may be evidenced by cervical enlargement with a variable alteration in echotexture. At this stage, the tumour may be mistaken for a cervical fibroid. It must be remembered that colposcopy is the diagnostic investigation for suspected cervical neoplasia and ultrasound has no role in the

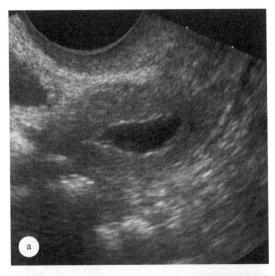

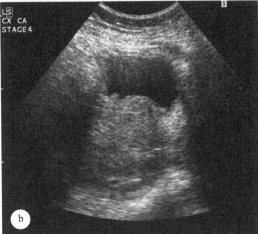

Figure 4.31 (a) Hydrometra: fluid is seen within the uterine cavity with a thin and regular endometrium. (b) Lower-segment transabdominal scan of a stage 4 cervical carcinoma.

detection of cervical malignancy outside of the fortuitous investigation of the symptomatic patient with per vaginam bleeding.

Irregularity of the cervical margin suggests parametrial invasion. Generally the uterine body and endometrial canal will appear normal. However, when cervical stenosis results from tumour infiltration of the cervical canal, an obstruction of the cervical canal and endometrial cavity may result in a collection of fluid (Fig. 4.31). Usually the amount of fluid

Table 4.6 Causes of cervical stenosis

Malignancy	Cervical carcinoma
	Endometrial carcinoma
Iatrogenic	Cone biopsy
	Post-radiotherapy
	Obstetric trauma
Postmenopausal atrophy	
Benign uterocervical pathology	Polyp
	Fibroid

in the cervical canal is small, although more significant collections may occur in the uterine cavity and a pyometra or haematometra may develop (Fig. 4.32). Regional lymphadenopathy may be apparent with enlarged pelvic lymph nodes being best visualised transvaginally. The examination should be extended to the upper abdomen in order to visualise the kidneys to check for hydronephrosis. The para-aortic area should be examined for lymphadenopathy and the liver examined for metastatic disease.

Hydrometra and pyometra may be seen at the time of diagnosis, post-treatment or, in the elderly patient, often many years after the successful treatment of the disease. Fluid collects in the uterine cavity due to chronic cervical narrowing either from radiation fibrosis or age-related stenosis. Advanced primary or recurrent disease may present with haematuria and urinary symptoms and ultrasound may show evidence of bladder invasion by the tumour (Fig. 4.33).

MRI is the investigation that defines tumour bulk, spread and recurrence most effectively, although ultrasound can be used to monitor renal dilatation.

Cervical stenosis

The causes of cervical stenosis are varied (Table 4.6) and a good clinical history is often required in order to elucidate the cause. However, whatever the cause, the clinical picture and the ultrasound appearance are likely to be similar. When obstruction allows

Figure 4.32 (a) Scan showing echogenic fluid within the uterine cavity in a tender uterus. (b) Haematometra – blood and clots are seen in the endometrial cavity.
(c) Hydronephrosis as a result of obstruction of the ureter in the pelvis.

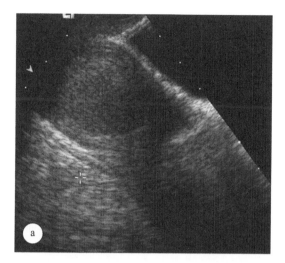

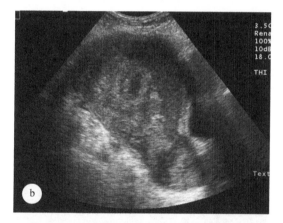

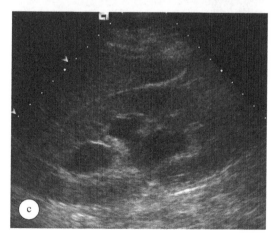

Figure 4.32

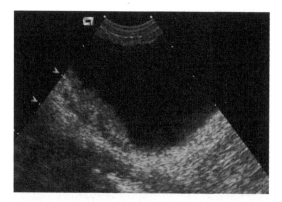

Figure 4.33 Thickened, abnormal bladder mucosa in malignant involvement of the bladder from carcinoma of the cervix.

Table 4.7 Uterine fluid collections

Infancy and childhood	Hydro/haematometrocolpos
Physiological	Menstruation
	Postmenopausal
Pregnancy	Normal early pregnancy
	Ectopic
	Haemorrhage
Retained products of conception	
Post-instrumentation	
Cervical stenosis (see above)	
Intrauterine pathology	Endometrial carcinoma
	Endometrial hyperplasia
	Endometrial polyp
Pelvic inflammatory disease	Endometritis

a significant amount of fluid to collect within the endometrial cavity, according to the type of fluid, the appearance is variously named as follows:

- hydrometra: serous fluid
- haematometra: blood
- pyometra: pus

In the case of pyometra, if gas-forming organisms are the cause of infection, then gas may be seen in the uterine cavity. In pyometra the uterus will be tender and the patient may have symptoms of infection, although chronic infections are often asymptomatic.

It must be remembered that a small amount of fluid seen in the postmenopausal uterus is normal as a result of atrophic cervical stenosis. This fluid can be useful in defining the endometrium (Fig. 4.34).

Uterine/endometrial fluid
The causes of fluid in the endometrial cavity may be physiological or pathological (Table 4.7)

Ultrasound appearances When there is fluid in the uterus it may be enlarged, with a distended endometrial cavity. The cervical canal may also be distended with fluid. The fluid may contain internal echoes, debris or fluid–fluid levels or gas.

An associated tumour mass may be apparent, for example endometrial, outlined by fluid.

Dilation of the cervical canal is a relatively straightforward procedure which will allow drainage of

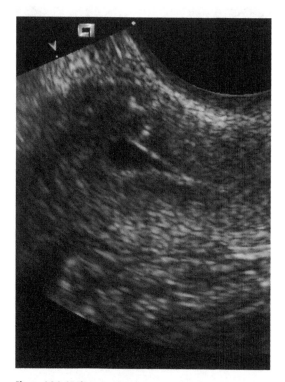

Figure 4.34 Hydrometra in a postmenopausal uterus – a normal finding.

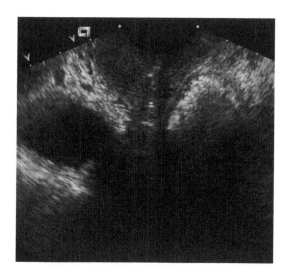

Figure 4.35 Air in the vagina.

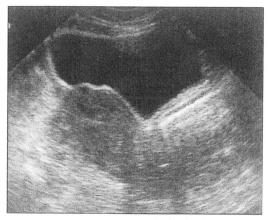

Figure 4.36 Sagittal image showing the strong reflection from a tampon in the vagina.

the abnormal fluid. However, where malignancy is involved, further investigations will be required.

The vagina

Vaginal pathology is generally recognised and investigated clinically. However, vaginal abnormalities are often diagnosed coincidentally at ultrasound examination, generally transabdominally as the vagina is not as well-visualised transvaginally due to its close proximity to the probe. Perineal examination may be more appropriate.

Ultrasound has a significant role to play in the investigation of congenital abnormalities (see Chapter 8).

Ultrasound can be useful in the investigation of retained tampons or other foreign bodies, although MRI is often required to assess these further, particularly in the paediatric age group.

Air may be visible in the vagina following instrumentation or sexual intercourse. This has the typical appearance of gas and is seen as flashing brightly echogenic foci in the upper vaginal vault (Fig. 4.35) and may indeed outline the cervix as seen in axial section. Similarly, an air-containing tampon may be visualised in the vagina transabdominally at ultra-

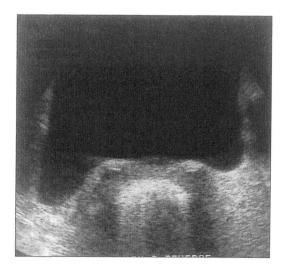

Figure 4.37 Transverse scan through the vagina showing a vaginal ring pessary, with strong acoustic shadowing.

sound as a strongly reflective lower structure producing acoustic shadowing (Fig. 4.36).

A vaginal pessary used in the treatment of uterine prolapse will be readily identified transabdominally. The superior and inferior margins of the ring are seen in the upper vagina on a sagittal section and the two lateral margins of the ring are seen in an axial plane. The ring will produce strong acoustic shadowing (Fig. 4.37).

Vaginal fluid collections

A small collection of fluid is not an uncommon finding at transabdominal ultrasound. This is most commonly seen at the time of menstruation. In a small child, small amounts of urine may occasionally be visualised following micturition. In the adult, urinary incontinence, a urinary fistula or an ectopically sited ureter may result in urine pooling in the vagina. Occasionally, extravaginal fluid collections such as paravaginal haematoma or urethral cyst may compress the vagina and give the erroneous impression of a vaginal fluid collection.

Haematocolpos Obstruction of the vagina will allow collection of fluid within. This usually occurs in young women post-menarche whereby the monthly menstrual blood collects in the vagina due to the lack of exit. The obstruction may lie distally at the level of the introitus, due to an imperforate hymen, or may result from a more proximal vaginal atresia, stenosis or the presence of a vaginal septum. These patients generally present with cyclical low abdomimal pain and amenorrhoea, lasting for some years after the expected date of the menarche. A lower abdominal mass may also be present. A similar condition is sometimes seen in infants or young children and, indeed, has been diagnosed antenatally. In this group of patients, the influence of the maternal hormones may be partially responsible for the condition (see Chapter 8).

When haematocolpos is associated with an anomaly of the genital tract, a thorough examination of the urinary tract is essential as in approximately a third of cases renal anomalies may be present. Unilateral renal agenesis or renal ectopia is the most likely anomaly to be found.

Ultrasound appearances A medium to large-sized cystic mass may be seen lying centrally in the lower abdomen. It should generally be possible to demonstrate continuity with the uterus and, indeed, the fluid may outline the ectocervix (Fig. 4.38). The mass has a thin wall and may contain fine internal echoes due to presence of altered blood. The appearance of

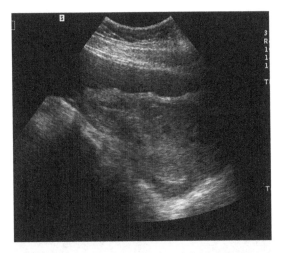

Figure 4.38 Fluid and blood clots distend the vagina in haematocolpos.

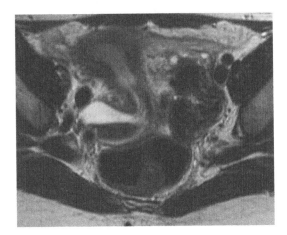

Figure 4.39 Magnetic resonance imaging scan showing haematocolpos.

the fluid may be very similar to that of an endometriotic cyst. Translabial ultrasound may be of value in demonstrating the length of the stenotic segment from the introitus.[28] MRI is also of value in this situation, with the information obtained allowing for accurate planning of reconstructive surgery (Fig. 4.39).

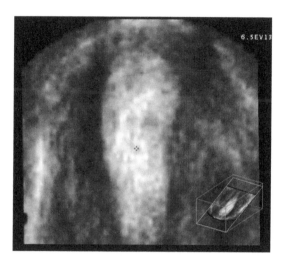
6.5EV13

Figure 4.40 Three-dimensional ultrasound image demonstrating the endometrium.

Three-dimensional (3D) ultrasound
The role of 3D in gynaecology has yet to be established but is increasingly used, in particular to define the shape and volume of the endometrium in three dimensions (Fig. 4.40).[29] However, MRI remains superior and therefore the use of 3D is more likely in situations when access to MRI is limited.

REFERENCES

1. F. Hasan, K. Arumugam and V. Sivanesaratnam, Uterine leiomyomota in pregnancy. *International Journal of Gynaecology and Obstetrics*, **34** (1991), 45–8.

2. R. E. Pelsang, J. Sorosky and T. Woods, Sonographic evaluation of the broad ligament of the uterus. *Journal of Clinical Ultrasound*, **27** (1999), 402–4.

3. W. M. Christopherson, E. O. Williamson and L. O. Gray, Leiomyosarcoma of the uterus. *Cancer*, **29** (1972), 1512–17.

4. L. G. Shapeero and H. Hrick, Mixed Müllerian sarcoma of the uterus: MR imaging findings. *American Journal of Radiology*, **153** (1989), 317–19.

5. S. H. Kim, H. Y. Hwang and B. I. Choi, Case report: uterine metastasis from stomach cancer: radiological findings. *Clinical Radiology*, **42** (1990), 285–6.

6. A. Malatsky, K. L. Reuter and B. Woda, Sonographic findings in primary uterine cervical lymphoma. *Journal of Clinical Ultrasound*, **19** (1991), 62–4.

7. W. H. Su, P. H. Wang, S. P. Chang and M. C. Su, Preoperative diagnosis of uterine lipoleiomyomata using ultrasound and computed tomography a case report. *European Journal of Gynaecology and Oncology*, **22** (2001), 439–40.

8. J. K. Gupta, P. F. W. Chien, D. Voit *et al.*, Ultrasonographic endometrial thickness for diagnosing endometrial pathology in women with postmenopausal bleeding: a meta analysis. *Acta Obstetrica Gynecologica Scandinavica*, **81** (2002), 799–816.

9. E. Epstein and L. Valentin, Managing women with post menopausal bleeding. *Best Practice in Research Clinic in Obstetrics and Gynaecology*, **18** (2004), 125–43.

10. Scottish Intercollegiate Guidelines Network Investigation of Post-menopausal Bleeding (2002).

11. American College of Obstetrics and Gynecologist Technology Assessment, Saline infusion sonography. *Journal of Gynaecology and Obstetrics*, **84** (2004), 95–8.

12. T. J. Dubinsky, K. Stroehlein, Y. Abu-ghazzeh, H. R. Parvey and N. Maklad, Prediction of benign and malignant disease: hysterosonographic-pathologic correlation. *Radiology*, **210** (1999), 393–7.

13. S. Laifer-Narin, N. Ragavendra, E. K. Parmenter and E. G. Grant, False-normal appearance of the endometrium on conventional transvaginal sonography: comparison with saline hyterosonography. *American Journal of Roentgenology*, **178** (2002), 129–33.

14. A. M. Darwish, A. M. Makhlouf, A. A. Youssof and H. A. Gadalla, Hysteroscopic myometrial biopsy in unexplained abnormal uterine bleeding. *European Journal of Obstetrics, Gynecology and Reproductive Biology*, **86** (1999), 139–43.

15. M. C. Anderson, E. B. Butler and G. V. P. Chamberlain, Oestrogen replacement and endometrial cancer. A statement by the British Cancer Group, *Lancet*, **I** (1981), 1359–60.

16. L. E. Rutqvist, H. Johansson, T. Signomklao *et al.*, Adjuvant tamoxifen therapy for early stage breast cancer and second primary malignancies. *Journal of the National Cancer Institute*, **87** (1995), 645–51.

17. A. Ayiomamitis, The epidemiology of cancer of the uterine corpus in Canada 1950–85. *International Journal of Gynaecology and Obstetrics*, **27** (1988), 205–11.

18. M. Berliere, A. Charles, C. Galant and J. Donnez, Uterine side effects of tamoxifen: a need for systematic pretreatment screening. *Obstetrics and Gynaecology*, **91** (1998), 40–4.

19. S. Cecchini, S. Ciatto, R. Bonardi *et al.*, Risk of endometrial cancer in breast cancer patients under long term adjuvant treatment with Tamoxifen. *Tumori*, **84** (1998), 21–3.

20. X. De Muylder, P. Neven, M. De Somer *et al.*, Endometrial lesions in patients undergoing tamoxifen therapy. *International Journal of Gynecology and Obstetrics*, **36** (1991), 127–30.

21. L. E. Hann, C. M. Kim, M. Gonen *et al.*, Sonohysterography compared with endometrial biopsy for evaluation of endoemtrium in tamoxifen treated women. *Obstetrics and Gynaecology Survey*, **59** (2004), 440–1.

22. N. J. Sebire, G. Makrydimaas, N. J. Agnantis, N. Zagorianakou and H. Rees, Updated diagnostic criteria for partial and complete hydatidiform mole in early pregnancy. *Anticancer Research*, **23** (2003), 1723–8.

23. B. W. Hancock and J. A. Tidy, Current management of molar pregnancy. *Journal of Reproductive Medicine*, **47** (2002), 347–54.

24. L. Savelli, G. Pilu, B. Valeri and L. Bovicelli, Transvaginal sonographic appearances of anaerobic endometris. *Ultrasound in Obstetrics and Gynaecology*, **21** (2003), 624–5.

25. R. Devlieger, T. D'Hoogle and D. Timmerman, Uterine adenomyosis in the infertility clinic. *Human Reproduction Update*, **9** (2003), 139–47.

26. E. Confino, J. Friberg, R. V. Giglia and N. Fleicher, Sonographic imaging of intrauterine adhesions. *Obstetrics and Gynecology*, **66** (1985), 596–8.

27. M. Cobby, J. Browning, A. Jones, E. Whipp and P. Goddard, Magnetic resonance imaging, computed tomography and endosonography in the local staging of carcinoma of the cervix. *British Journal of Radiology*, **63** (1990), 673–9.

28. K. A. Scanlon, M. A. Pozniak, M. Fagerholm and S. Shapiro, Value of transperineal sonography in the assessment of vaginal atresia. *American Journal of Roentgenology*, **154** (1990), 545–8.

29. R. Salim, B. Woelfer, M. Backos, L. Regan and D. Jurkovic, Reproducibility of three dimensional ultrasound diagnosis of congenital uterine anomalies. *Ultrasound in Obstetrics and Gynecology*, **21** (2003), 578–82.

BIBLIOGRAPHY

J. Anderson, *Gynaecologic Imaging* (Churchill Livingstone, 1999).

S. Robby, M. C. Anderson and P. Russell, *Pathology of the Female Reproductive Tract* (Churchill Liuingstone, 2002).

A. C. Fleischer, F. A. Manning, P. Jeanty and R. Romero, *Sonography in Obstetric and Gynaecology* (Prentice Hall International)

5

Pathology of the ovaries, fallopian tubes and adnexae

Damian J. M. Tolan and Michael J. Weston

St James's University Hospital, Leeds

Introduction

Ultrasound has become an essential part of the gynaecological evaluation of the adnexae (which comprise the ovaries, fallopian tubes and broad ligament). In this chapter we will discuss the pathology, ultrasound imaging features and aspects of management of a range of conditions affecting the adnexae and conditions that may mimic adnexal pathology. We will concentrate on important or common conditions, with particular emphasis on the ovaries.

Clinical presentation

Patients referred for ultrasound examination of the pelvis may present with a range of symptoms. *Pain* is common and may be related to ovulation (mittelschmerz), menstruation (particularly in endometriosis) or intercourse (dyspareunia). Chronic pain may indicate pelvic inflammatory disease (PID) and acute severe pain may herald an emergency in the form of ovarian torsion or ectopic pregnancy. However some women complain of *pressure* rather than pain, often related to masses causing compression and displacement of pelvic organs. The close proximity of the adnexae to other organs may produce *gastrointestinal* or *renal tract symptoms*, which may misdirect the clinical evaluation away from the real cause for the complaint. *Bloating*

and *distension*, though non-specific, are symptoms that may suggest ascites or massive ovarian tumours.

Alteration to the normal *menstrual cycle*, with irregular bleeding or amenorrhoea, and *infertility* or *subfertility* are further indicators of ovarian pathology ranging from polycystic ovary syndrome (PCOS) to hormone-secreting tumours.

Increasingly, with improvement in technology and increase in the demand for examinations, pathology is being discovered incidentally on imaging examinations for unrelated complaints. This emphasises the point that important ovarian pathology is often *asymptomatic* and helps to explain why ovarian cancer is known as the silent killer, resulting from the late presentation of many cases and the apparent lack of symptoms in the early phase of disease.

Essential patient details

Prior to scanning the patient should be interviewed to discuss her presenting symptoms and to obtain information essential to the correct interpretation of the scan. This should include the following details:

- patient's age – as adnexal masses in premenarchal or older postmenopausal women are more likely to be malignant
- date of the first day of the last period and normal length of cycle
- menstrual status (premenarchal, pre- or postmenopausal)

- medications (including hormone replacement, oral or depot contraceptives and tamoxifen)
- gynaecological history, including previous operations

Acceptability of transvaginal scanning should be ensured in an appropriate setting prior to scanning.

Benign physiological (functional) cysts

Cyst formation in the ovary is a normal consequence of ovarian function. These physiological cysts arise from the hormone-regulated development of follicles within the ovary. Larger cysts result from physiological over-stimulation of a dominant graafian follicle and are a cause of concern because they may mimic more serious pathology.

Follicular cysts

These are the commonest clinically detectable ovarian masses and one of the most common causes of an ovarian mass on ultrasound. They arise within an ovary because of a failure of the mature Graafian follicle to rupture and release the ovum. Typically, rupture occurs when the follicles reach 2.5 cm in diameter. However follicular cysts continue to grow under hormone mediation and may reach up to 8–10 cm in diameter in some cases.

The typical appearance is of a unilocular cyst over 3 cm in diameter with a thin, smooth wall and echo-free fluid within it (Fig. 5.1). Some normal cysts may undergo haemorrhagic change, producing echogenic fluid.[1] The normal history is of spontaneous regression within 4–6 weeks. A repeat examination is recommended in 5–7 weeks to ensure resolution of the follicle – a malignant cyst will not regress in size.

Corpus luteum cysts

The corpus luteum is formed by rupture of the mature graafian follicle. Its function is to produce progesterone and oestrogens to support early pregnancy in the period before the placenta takes over

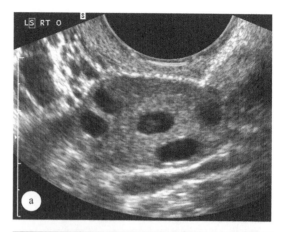

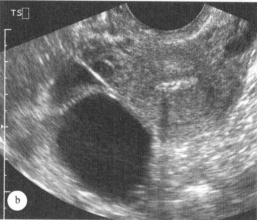

Figure 5.1 (a) Normal ovary showing a few small follicular structures. (b) A simple follicular cyst of the ovary. There are no internal echoes.

this role. When these follicles fail to involute, cysts are formed.

The clinical picture may be pain with delayed menses or amenorrhoea. In this setting the most important differential is ectopic pregnancy: this may mimic the imaging findings of a haemorrhagic corpus luteum, particularly as there is often associated endometrial proliferation. Knowledge of the result of a pregnancy test is advantageous. Clearly a well-demonstrated intrauterine pregnancy would support an adnexal lesion being a corpus luteum, but an important exception is in the setting of in

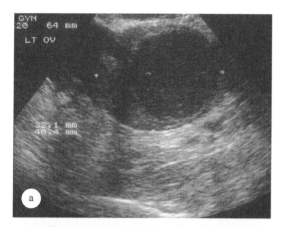

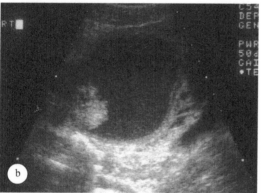

Figure 5.2 (a) A small luteal cyst of the ovary showing uniform internal echoes due to recent haemorrhage. (b) A large luteal cyst showing internal echoes due to haemorrhage as well as a focal lump due to clot retraction.

vitro fertilisation (IVF) where multiple pregnancy and ectopic pregnancy are commoner than in the general population and rarely both may coexist (i.e. heterotopic pregnancy).

The sonographic findings of a corpus luteum cyst are variable. Typically these cysts are hypoechoic with thick walls and may vary in size from 2 to 10 cm, although most are less than 3 cm in diameter. Haemorrhage is often present, resulting in the appearance of either a complex cystic mass containing fluid with internal echoes or a solid adnexal structure (Fig. 5.2). Occasionally layering of contents may occur. The Doppler and colour flow characteristics are non-specific and vary as the corpus luteum matures and involutes but peripheral diastolic flow is normal in these cysts during the luteal phase of the cycle. Corpus luteum cysts can cause complications through rupture and haemorrhage, obstructed delivery and by undergoing torsion. A persistent large corpus in the second half of pregnancy may require surgical excision to prevent later complications. Similarly, a complex haemorrhagic luteal cyst may simulate malignancy. In this setting follow-up scanning is needed to ensure reduction or resolution.

Parovarian cysts (fimbral cysts, peritoneal inclusion cysts)

While these are not truly ovarian, they may mimic ovarian cysts and so are dealt with in this section of the chapter. Parovarian cysts arise in the broad ligament, originating either from the peritoneum covering the ligament or embryological remnants of the wolffian ducts that run from the vaginal vestibule to the ovary within the ligament. They comprise up to 10% of adnexal masses, tending to affect premenopausal women, and are seen separate from the neighbouring ovary. Cysts are fluid-filled and thin-walled with no septations or internal soft-tissue projections.[2] In common with ovarian cysts they may be complicated by haemorrhage, torsion and rupture and can reach several centimetres in diameter, extending out of the pelvis.[3] Peritoneal inclusion cysts are more likely to be seen if there has been prior surgery. The cyst walls will conform to adjacent structures and often show acute angular margins as a characteristic feature. Not all pelvic cysts arise from gynaecological structures. Sometimes intestinal lesions may mimic an ovarian lesion. Carefully assessing if the lesion is attached to bowel will avoid this pitfall, though a precise diagnosis may only be made confidently following surgery (Fig. 5.3).

Postmenopausal cysts

Simple cysts of less than 5 cm in size are a very common finding in postmenopausal women during pelvic ultrasound examination. It is important to

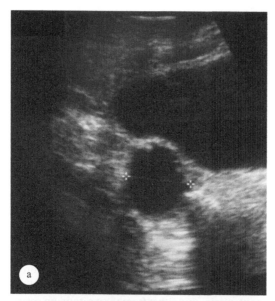

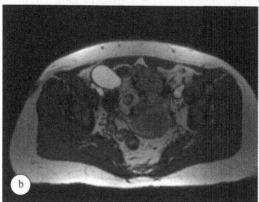

Figure 5.3 (a) Ultrasound image showing a simple pelvic cyst. This was at first thought to be ovarian, but the ovary was separate to this. (b) Magnetic resonance image of the same lesion. Its elongated oval shape is more apparent. This lesion was found to be a mucocele of the appendix at surgery.

understand that these cysts do not equate to cancer and will not become cancerous. The difficulty arises because very occasionally (in less than 1% of cases) an ovarian cancer will present features indistinguishable from a simple cyst. Over 50% of postmenopausal simple cysts will resolve within 4 months of the initial assessment, though some will persist unchanged for

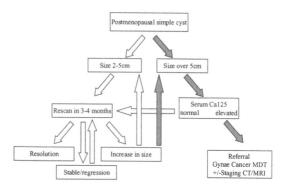

Figure 5.4 Flowchart demonstrating management of postmenopausal cysts.

a very long time. We have constructed a flow chart (Fig. 5.4) for the management of these patients to try to prevent inappropriate over-investigation, based on Royal College of Obstetricians and Gynaecologists guidelines.[4] Ideally, a decision on whether to operate or to ignore the cyst can be achieved without more than three sequential scans. Continuing to follow up a simple postmenopausal cyst for longer than this becomes indistinguishable from offering ovarian cancer screening.

Congenital cysts

These are most often discovered incidentally during prenatal and neonatal ultrasound examination and are probably due to follicular stimulation by maternal hormones. They are seldom clinically significant and the natural history is of spontaneous resolution. Rarely, surgery is required either for torsion or for large cysts causing problems due to mass effect, resulting in compression of adjacent viscera and splinting of the diaphragm.[5]

Benign ovarian pathology

Polycystic ovary syndrome

This is a common complex endocrine disorder affecting 5–10% of women. It presents with menstrual disturbance, obesity and hyperandrogenism

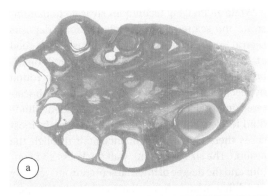

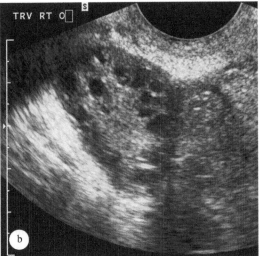

Figure 5.5 (a) Histological specimen of a polycystic ovary. This shows the typical features one would expect to see on ultrasound of numerous small follicles and an increase in stroma. (b) An ultrasound image of a polycystic ovary showing the same features.

resulting from testosterone and androstenedione production, which leads to increased hair growth (hirsutism). The criteria for ultrasound diagnosis of PCOS have recently been revised in the light of improved ultrasound technology and better understanding of the condition.[6] The diagnosis can be supported when one or more of the following features are demonstrated (Fig. 5.5):

• 12 or more follicles (3–12 mm diameter) are present in an ovary (either peripheral or diffusely arranged)

• ovarian volume is over 10 ml/s (when no follicles measuring over 10 mm in diameter are present)

Only a single ovary need be affected to make the diagnosis. If a large follicle is present (over 10 mm), then the volume should be calculated on a repeat scan when the ovary is quiescent to prevent overestimation of ovarian volume. Bright ovarian stroma relative to the myometrium is no longer an essential part of the diagnosis but is specific to the condition and provides supporting evidence in the presence of the essential features above. This appearance is thought by some authorities to be caused by increased sound transmission through follicles in the ovaries.

The appearance of a polycystic ovary is much commoner than the diagnosis of the syndrome. An important point emphasised in these new diagnostic guidelines is that imaging findings alone should not diagnose PCOS in an asymptomatic patient. In this situation the possibility may be raised but further supporting evidence in terms of the patient's history, clinical examination and blood tests (elevated androgens and luteinising hormone with low/normal follicle-stimulating hormone level) should be obtained before a firm diagnosis is made.[6]

Endometriosis

This is a relatively common condition, affecting around 5–10% of all women but accounting for a high proportion of patients presenting with infertility problems and chronic pelvic pain. It is thought to arise from deposits of endometrial tissue seeding outside the uterus during retrograde menstruation (i.e. along the fallopian tubes into the peritoneum). Classically symptoms are cyclical, occurring during menstruation when ectopic endometrial deposits bleed, but intermenstrual bleeding and menorrhagia may occur. Interestingly, the bulk of disease does not appear to correlate closely with symptoms; those with large-volume disease are sometimes asymptomatic, while those with relatively minor deposits on imaging and laparoscopy may have severe intractable symptoms.

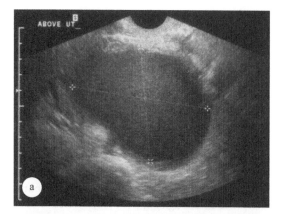

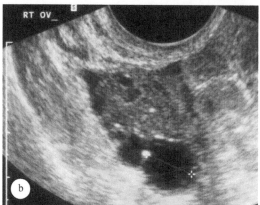

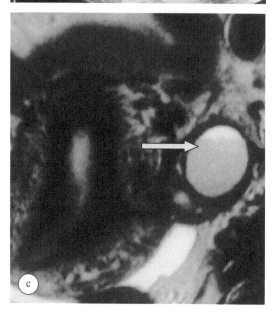

While all imaging techniques struggle to demonstrate the scattered small endometriosis deposits seen at times during laparoscopy, ultrasound is good at demonstrating focal masses called endometriomas. They are usually thin-walled ovoid or round hypoechoic masses, and may contain fluid with scattered internal echoes or gravity-dependent fluid–fluid levels from layering of haemorrhage. In most cases there is acoustic enhancement through the lesion.[7] The size (1–20 cm), wall thickness and contour and the degree of internal septation are variable and differentiation from other pelvic pathology, particularly ovarian malignancy, is often impossible. In this setting magnetic resonance imaging (MRI) is an extremely useful tool; the unique signal characteristics of endometrioma produce high signal (bright) on T1-weighted images, with no loss of signal on fat-saturated T1-weighted sequences and intermediate or low signal areas on T2, due to the blood products within it[8] (Fig. 5.6). This allows differentiation in most cases from dermoid tumours, which normally contain fat, and ovarian carcinoma, and helps avoid unnecessary surgery.

An important consideration in cases of endometriosis is the distribution of disease. Most often deposits are found in gravity-dependent areas within the pelvis, involving the ovaries, rectosigmoid colon[9] and urinary bladder.[10] The disease is also recognised to occur at the site of caesarean-section scar.[11] Transvaginal and transrectal scans are very sensitive methods of assessing plaque-like deposits of endometriosis along the uterosacral ligaments by demonstrating thickening of the rectovaginal septum and uterosacral ligaments.[12] Disease may also disseminate to other sites in the abdomen, spreading along peritoneal recesses to involve other

---

Figure 5.6 Endometriosis (a) A large endometrioma showing the typical uniform low-level internal echoes on ultrasound. (b) Tiny cystic endometriotic deposits around the surface of an ovary. There is a fleck of associated calcification. (c) Magnetic resonance of an endometriotic cyst. Layering of the signal intensity is seen from the blood within the cyst (arrow).

sections of bowel and even across the diaphragm to involve the pleural space.

Torsion

Ovarian torsion normally presents in the first three decades of life with a short history of acute-onset lower abdominal pain, often localised to one side, and accompanied by nausea and vomiting. Fever and elevated white cell counts are not commonly present.[13,14] Intermittent pain may precede the acute event, weeks or months before diagnosis, due to intermittent torsion of the ovary.

Patients are predisposed to torsion by coexisting ovarian pathology, such as follicular cysts, but in many cases there is no underlying abnormality present. The process of torsion of the vascular pedicle causes venous outflow obstruction and engorgement of the ovary. Eventually gangrene ensues, as a result of either venous infarction or arterial occlusion.

The diagnosis is suggested by unilateral enlargement of a rounded or oval-shaped ovary containing multiple enlarged follicles, although these follicles are not always present. The ovarian stroma is often brighter than adjacent myometrium and free fluid may be present in the pelvis. The mass may be solid with posterior acoustic enhancement or cystic.[13,14] Free fluid is present in the majority of cases. Rarely patients may present with massive ovarian enlargement, which can be bilateral, mimicking neoplasia[15] (Fig. 5.7). A further indicator of torsion is that the ovary may lie in an abnormal position in the midline behind the uterus. A peripheral blood flow pattern may be present but colour flow can be absent in infarction. Importantly, normal colour flow does not exclude the diagnosis, which may occur in cases of intermittent torsion.

This is often an underdiagnosed condition sonographically and clinicians with a high index of suspicion should not be falsely reassured by a normal scan. In this setting laparoscopy is required to ensure that the ovaries are healthy and, if torted, detorsion and fixation performed or oophorectomy in the presence of gangrene.

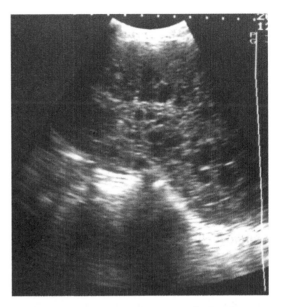

Figure 5.7 Massive ovarian oedema as a result of ovarian torsion.

Ovarian hyperstimulation

This arises most often as a result of ovarian hormone stimulation in infertility techniques such as prior to egg-harvesting in IVF. It may also occur in single or multiple pregnancies, hydatidiform mole and choriocarcinoma.[16,17] Briefly, the findings consist of enlarged ovaries where increasing diameter correlates with disease severity (from 5 cm in grade 2 to over 12 cm in grades 5 and 6). Multiple large cysts are present and there may be associated ascites and pleural effusions. This is dealt with more fully in Chapter 7.

Absent ovaries and ovarian remnant syndrome

Either or both ovaries are sometimes not visualised during assessment of the pelvis, particularly when only a transabdominal scan is performed. It is important to remember that some patients may have no ovaries at all. This should be considered particularly in cases of amenorrhoea. Turner's syndrome, where only one X chromosome is present, may result in absent ovaries. Patients have short stature and may have associated renal and skeletal developmental anomalies. Swyer's syndrome results in isolated absence of the ovaries without other abnormality.

Ovarian remnant syndrome presents in patients who have had previous incomplete oophorectomy with abdominal pain and sometimes a palpable mass. The residual functioning ovarian tissue hypertrophies to become an enlarged multicystic structure and haemorrhage is often present. The mass may cause ureteric obstruction and hydronephrosis.[18] An ovarian mass can be present when the ovaries are expected to be absent.

Multimodality and multidisciplinary assessment of ovarian tumours

Any case of possible ovarian malignancy requires multidisciplinary assessment by a team with experienced gynaecologists, pathologists, radiologists and oncologists. This serves two purposes: to decide, first, on what further investigations are required, and second, what treatments should be offered with a view to cure or palliation of symptoms.

Preoperative biopsy should not be done to confirm the diagnosis of localised ovarian malignancy. It is contraindicated because of the risk of seeding tumour into the peritoneum and upstaging the patient from early stage I to stage II or III with a subsequent poorer prognosis. Likewise, drainage of ascites is best avoided if surgery is planned in the near future anyway. Occasionally there are reports of unwary clinicians inserting drainage catheters into ovarian cysts in the mistaken belief they are draining either ascites or the bladder. Tumour markers are not always helpful, with CA125 elevated in only 50% of stage I tumours. MRI scanning has a useful role in the evaluation of indeterminate lesions on ultrasound. Many benign lesions have characteristic features on MR that allow differentiation from ovarian carcinoma. In the case of ovarian cancers, an assessment of the stage of local disease can be made with greater confidence on MRI and the ultrasound features of the tumour confirmed. This is particularly helpful in borderline cases on ultrasound, where MRI

allows a more complete characterisation of the lesion in question. Computed tomography (CT) scanning has a role in the staging assessment of disseminated disease, where there is no doubt about the malignant features on ultrasound or where metastatic disease has been demonstrated on the ultrasound scan. Neither technique can assess the peritoneum well for small-volume metastases, although delayed MRI following gadolinium is producing some promising results. Laparoscopy gives the best evaluation in these circumstances.

Imaging allows preoperative planning of the type of surgery required, with radical hysterectomy, bilateral oophorectomy and omentectomy as the standard curative technique for ovarian cancer (*the big operation*). This compares with much more limited surgery in benign or some borderline malignant cases, where unilateral oophorectomy or cystectomy may be considered (*the small operation*). In cases of disseminated disease where radical surgical debulking is inappropriate, imaging-guided biopsy of peritoneal deposits is a simple and effective method of obtaining histological confirmation of the diagnosis, and can assist in planning palliative chemotherapy for symptom control. In some cases, where there is inoperable malignancy on initial scanning, some patients may proceed, after a confirmatory biopsy, to chemotherapy to down-stage the ovarian tumour before interval debulking surgery. It is important to have confirmation of disseminated ovarian malignancy, rather than disseminated metastatic breast cancer, for example, as the treatment options are different and prognosis far more grave in the case of breast metastasis in this situation. Ultrasound has an additional role in facilitating periodic guided drainage for palliation of malignant ascites. This is very well tolerated by patients and provides excellent symptom relief.

Benign tumours – epithelial neoplasms

Serous cystadenoma

These are more common than mucinous cystadenomas and tend to affect younger women of

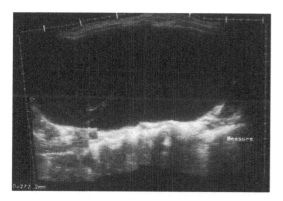

Figure 5.8 An extended field of view ultrasound used to show the full extent of this ovarian serous cystadenoma. There are a few fine septations present.

reproductive age and account for between 20 and 50% of all ovarian neoplasms. They are often smaller than benign mucinous tumours and bilateral lesions are much more common. Cysts have thin walls and are either unilocular or contain multiple thin septations (Fig. 5.8). Small (< 3 mm) internal papillary projections may be present. Internal fluid is usually echo-free but may be echogenic where haemorrhage has occurred. Once again, if there is rupture of the cyst, free fluid may be present and Doppler studies are not very helpful at distinguishing benign from malignant disease. Surgery is therefore often performed as primary treatment.

Mucinous cystadenomas

These are classically unilateral ovarian tumours presumed to arise from metaplasia of normal epithelial tissue. Women aged from 20 to 50 are the group most commonly affected but these tumours may occur at any age and they account for around 15% of all benign tumours. They consist of large and sometimes massive cysts (up to 50 cm) with thin walls and multiple thin-walled locules. They contain mucin, a thick proteinaceous fluid, which has an echogenic appearance on ultrasound, and distinct fluid–fluid levels are sometimes present (Fig. 5.9). Sonographic morphological criteria and Doppler interrogation alone cannot accurately predict benignity, and these

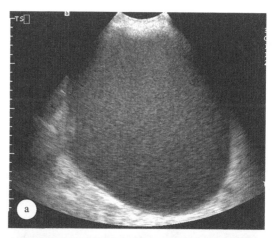

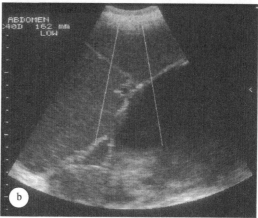

Figure 5.9 Mucinous cystadenoma. (a) A large unilocular cyst containing uniform low-level echoes. This can mimic the appearance of an endometrioma but the size and the clinical history should aid in the differentiation. Magnetic resonance would be able to distinguish these lesions if required. (b) A large multilocular cyst, with the locules displaying different levels of internal echo. The septa are thickened, increasing the level of concern for underlying malignancy.

lesions are removed to assess for malignant change and to prevent torsion and rupture.

Rupture of the mucinous contents of these tumours into the peritoneal cavity results in *pseudomyxoma peritonei*, a condition where mucinous collections are formed in the abdomen leading to distension, peritoneal thickening and mass effect on adjacent organs. This carries a poor prognosis due to

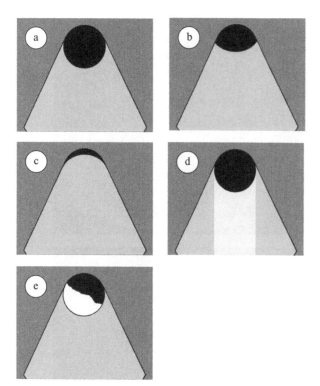

Figure 5.10 Line diagram indicating the differing features of dermoid tumours. (a) Hyperechoic mass with all the borders visible. (b) The distal borders are visible. (c) Only the proximal border is visible ('tip of the iceburg'). (d) Dense shadow behind mass. (e) Fat–fluid level.

its propensity to recur after surgery, which is the only effective treatment presently available. Pseudomyxoma pertonei is also associated with perforation of appendiceal epithelial tumours resulting in mucinous tumour dissemination on peritoneal surfaces.

Germ cell tumours – dermoid/teratoma

These are complex germ cell tumours most commonly presenting in younger women of reproductive age, but all age groups may be affected. They account for around 15% of all ovarian tumours and arise from ectodermal (hair, skin, sweat glands), mesodermal (bone, muscle and cartilage) and endodermal tissue

elements (neural tissue and vascular) in variable amounts. They are most commonly cystic but solid teratomas, although rare, are recognised. The differing proportion of fat, calcium, hair and soft-tissue components results in a highly variable appearance on ultrasound. A simple classification system, with a high predictive value, and based on sonographic features has been formulated as follows:[19]

- I: an echogenic mass of varying density and shadowing subdivided into:
  - A: all borders visible
  - B: distal border visible
  - C: only proximal border visible: 'tip of the iceberg'
- II: echogenic particles in a hypoechoic medium 'dermoid mesh'
- III: Cyst with fat–fluid level, where the uppermost oil layer is echo-free (Fig. 5.10)

A pathognomonic distinct hyperechoic mural nodule or 'dermoid plug' may also be present, representing an ingrowth of solid tissue, such as hair or teeth, from the tumour wall[20] (Fig. 5.11). Possible pitfalls in the diagnosis are, firstly, the potential for failing to recognise the presence of a dermoid because of similarity to the echogenic contents of bowel loops within the pelvis or, secondly, mistaking the hyperechogenicity of a small dermoid for fresh haemorrhage within a cyst.

Torsion is the commonest complication of these tumours but rupture may occur, usually related to pregnancy. Dermoids rarely undergo malignant degeneration (around 3%) in older women, but imaging cannot differentiate non-metastatic malignant from benign tumours. MRI is the best test to confirm the presence of fat and other mesenchymal components within the tumour; enhancing nodules are a cause for concern, suggesting malignancy.

Ovarian stromal tumours

Solid ovarian masses are relatively uncommon, accounting for about 5% of ovarian tumours. The differential of a solid adnexal mass, after a pedunculated uterine fibroid has been considered, should

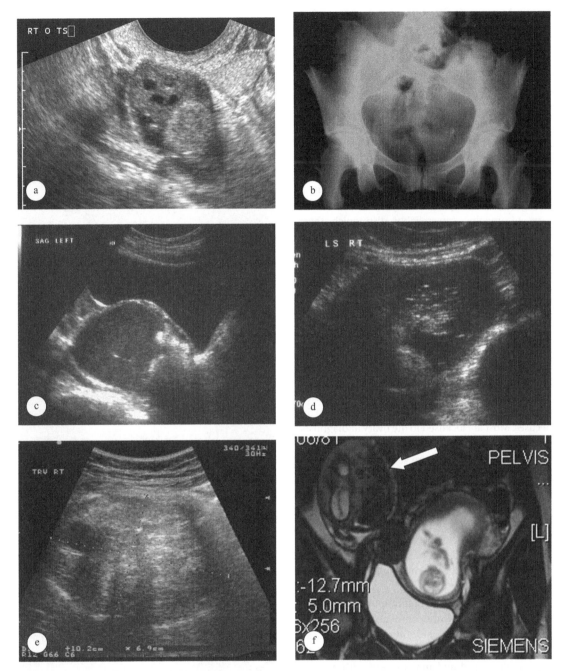

Figure 5.11 Several examples of dermoid tumours. (a) A small bright focus within an ovary. This could be either a small dermoid tumour or an area of haemorrhage. A follow-up ultrasound scan will tell the difference as an area of haemorrhage will resolve. (b) A plain radiograph of the pelvis. The air-filled tampon is seen to be displaced to the right by a fat-density left adnexal lesion. This lesion contains a tooth-like structure in its inferior aspect. (c) A dermoid showing the characteristic feature of an echogenic plug casting a dense echo shadow. (d) There is a collection of fine parallel lines within this dermoid. Another very typical feature. (e and f) An incidental adnexal mass found during pregnancy is confirmed on magnetic resonance imaging to be a dermoid. Magnetic resonance is particularly useful for characterising adnexal masses in pregnancy.

include the ovarian stromal tumours. The most commonly recognised sonographic appearance for all of these tumours is an isoechoic or hypoechoic mass with acoustic enhancement. However, beam attenuation may also occur in the tumour, resulting in acoustic shadows.[21] Foci of cystic degeneration with or without septations may be present, particularly in granulosa cell tumours;[22] and areas of calcification may be seen in fibromas.[23] No form of imaging can reliably distinguish these tumours; histological examination is the definitive investigation.

Thecomas are solid, fat-filled oestrogen-producing tumours occurring in perimenopausal and postmenopausal women. They are benign and account for around 1% of all ovarian tumours. The tumour-related hormone effects may result in postmenopausal bleeding or menorrhagia related to endometrial thickening and the presence of endometrial cancer is a well-recognised association.

Granulosa cell tumours are low-grade malignant hormone-secreting tumours and are bilateral in 5% of cases. Most are localised to the ovary at diagnosis, but recurrence after surgery occurs in up to 10% of cases, which may require sequential operations over a number of years to remove recurrent tumours. Patients are usually postmenopausal and the clinical presentation is identical to thecoma.

Sertoli–Leydig cell tumours produce androgens and oestrogens and are discovered in young women investigated for virilisation, usually in a search for polycystic ovaries. They are low-grade malignancies and are managed surgically.

Fibromas are benign stromal tumours of varying size (Fig. 5.12). They are composed, as the name suggests, of fibrous tissue, sometimes in association with hormonally active thecal cells. Patients are often middle-aged and may present with a mass, pain, menstrual disturbance or, less commonly, with ascites and right-sided pleural effusions, known as *Meig's syndrome*. Symptoms resolve completely following successful removal of the tumour. There may be marked overlap in the histological appearance of fibromas and thecomas, where they are termed fibrothecomas.

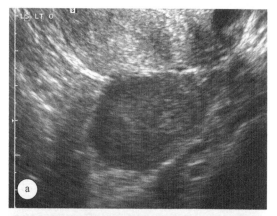

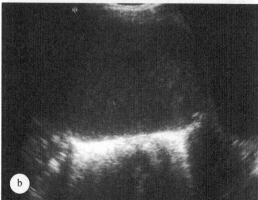

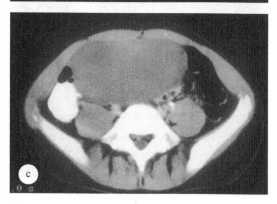

Figure 5.12 Ovarian fibromas. (a) A small fibroma within the ovary. (b and c) A much larger fibroma shown on both ultrasound and computed tomography scan. Note that there is posterior acoustic enhancement through this solid tumour. Imaging cannot reliably characterise a solid adnexal mass and surgery and histology are required to achieve a diagnosis. It may however be possible to avoid 'the big cancer operation'.

Brenner tumours may arise from ovarian stromal tissue or epithelium and are composed of fibrous tissue, similar to fibroma. They are rare and usually benign, although malignant forms are recognised. While most cases are not hormonally active, oestrogen-related side-effects have been seen in some cases and tumours can reach several centimetres in size.

Subserosal or pedunculated uterine fibroids

Although clearly not an ovarian neoplasm, uterine fibroids need to be mentioned in this section because of the problems they can pose in the diagnosis of ovarian neoplasms. Pedunculated fibroids can vary greatly in size and position within the pelvis, and typical imaging features of a homogeneous or heterogeneous solid mass with tissue characteristics ranging from hypo- to hyperechoic can be altered in the presence of necrosis of larger lesions, resulting in a more complex cystic appearance on ultrasound (Fig. 5.13). In this setting, a younger patient may unwittingly be diagnosed as having ovarian carcinoma, particularly when CT confirms the localised mass without the further tissue characterisation or detailed multiplanar examination available with MR scanning. Similarly, in older women, in whom fibroids are uncommon due to involution after the menopause, an ovarian tumour may be mistaken for a necrotic pedunculated fibroid. Clearly the management and counselling of the patient are very different for the two conditions. We would like to raise the readers' awareness of this potential pitfall and advise them to be extremely cautious in dismissing complex masses as pedunculated fibroids, particularly in the postmenopausal female, without full assessment, including MRI where appropriate.

Malignant ovarian tumours

Ovarian carcinoma

Epidemiology of ovarian cancer
Ovarian cancer is a significant health problem, being the fifth most common cancer in women and also the leading cause of death from gynaecological malignancies. In 1992, 4360 women died of ovarian cancer in the UK[24] and in 1994 in the USA there were approximately 13 600 deaths.[25] However, to place these large figures in perspective, the disease prevalence is between 30 and 50 cases per 100 000 population and the lifetime incidence is one in 70 women (in comparison, the lifetime risk of breast cancer is one in 12). It is uncommon in black women.[26] Most cases occur after the age of 45.

Survival depends on the stage of the disease at diagnosis. The early stages of the disease do not have any specific symptoms and so nearly 60% of women present with disease that has already spread with abdominal metastases such as in the omentum (stage III) or with distant metastases outside the peritoneal cavity (stage IV) to lung, liver, bone and distant lymph nodes. These women only have a one in 10 chance of surviving for 5 years. Conversely those women (25%) who present with the disease confined to the ovary (stage I) have a six or seven in 10 chance of surviving for the same period. Stage II disease with ovarian spread confined to the pelvis has an intermediate survival (Table 5.1).

Risk factors for ovarian cancer
The cause of ovarian cancer is not known, though there are women who are at higher risk than others. Risk factors include greater age, nulliparity, northern European or North American descent, and a family history of ovarian cancer. There is a theory that ovulation itself is a causative factor, as the risk of ovarian cancer appears to be decreased by pregnancy, breast-feeding and oral contraceptives, all of which suppress ovulation.

Women who have one close relative with ovarian cancer have a threefold increase in lifetime risk, whereas those with two close relatives have a dramatic increase to a 40% lifetime risk. As many as 5% of ovarian cancers occurring before the age of 50 may be due to familial cancer.[26] Mutations in the genes *BRCA1* and *2* may account for most of these families.[27] This raises the intriguing prospect of genetic testing to enable individuals to learn if they carry a cancer-predisposing mutation. Not all

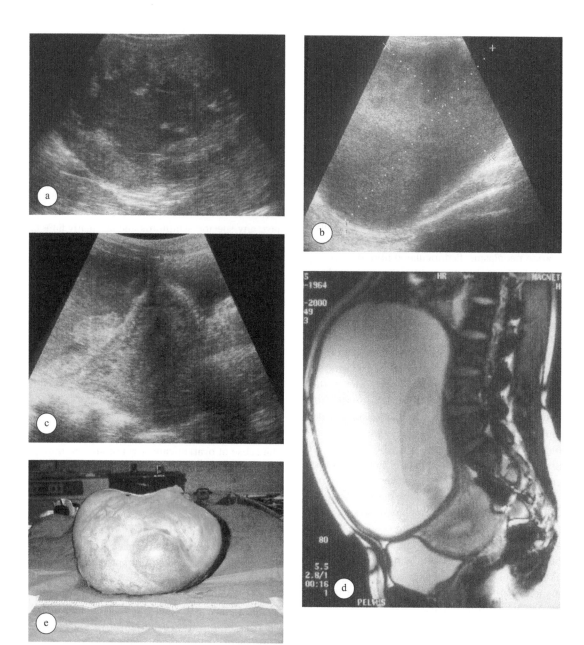

Figure 5.13 (a) Degenerating pedunculated fibroid. An adnexal lesion with central cavitation was identified during early pregnancy. (b and c) The pregnancy miscarried. The woman was seen several months later to have a large abdominal mass. Taken in isolation, these ultrasound images would be of concern because of the apparently nodular margins and because the lesion appears separate from the uterus. (d) Magnetic resonance shows the full extent of this adnexal mass. (e) A large, centrally cavitated fibroid is removed at surgery. This sequence of images shows the value of obtaining a history and comparing old images with new. The progression of the cavitation in a benign fibroid becomes apparent.

Table 5.1 Abbreviated International Federation of Gynecology and Obstetrics (FIGO) staging of ovarian carcinoma

Stage	Location	Symptoms
I	Confined to ovary	Asymptomatic
		Good prognosis after surgery
		Diagnosed by screening or during investigation for other symptomatic conditions
II	Spread confined to the pelvis	Usually asymptomatic, diagnosed as above
III	Abdominal metastases – omentum, lymphadenopathy – peritoneal implants, e.g. liver surface	Presents with abdominal enlargement or symptoms from distant metastases
		Poor 5-year survival
IV	Distant metastases – liver parenchyma, lungs	

those at risk want such testing, though those from a higher economic class and those with more relatives affected are more likely to request the test.[28] The implications of a positive test need to be explored fully before testing, including factors such as difficulties in obtaining a mortgage or life insurance. Furthermore, whether a positive genetic predisposition should lead to active ovary and breast screening or even prophylactic bilateral oophorectomy (and subcutaneous mastectomy) needs to be discussed.

Imaging features and scoring systems

Ultrasound has a very valuable role to play in the characterisation of adnexal masses. There are proponents for the use of various morphological, spectral and colour Doppler criteria both transabdominally and transvaginally in the differentiation of malignant from benign ovarian disease. *Morphological scoring systems* have been proposed by several authors.[29,30] They all have in common the association of malignancy with the presence of a large size (over 10 cm), a solid or partly solid content and papillae (Fig. 5.14). Fine septations and daughter cysts are associated with benignity. A review of these scoring systems found their sensitivities to range from 62 to 100%, the specificities from 73 to 95% and the positive predictive values from 31 to 83%. Using their own criteria they could obtain 100% sensitivity, but only at the cost of a low specificity of 37%.

This was caused by abscesses, teratomas and haemorrhagic cysts being indistinguishable from malignant tumours on appearance alone.

The low specificity of morphology prompted a search for *Doppler criteria* of malignancy. Initial reports of the use of resistance and pulsatility indices were very encouraging, but a series of later reports showed that spectral Doppler is not helpful because there is too great an overlap in the indices between benign and malignant disease.[31–34] With time, however, Doppler's true role, particularly colour Doppler, is becoming clearer. Buy and colleagues,[35] in their study of 132 adnexal masses in 115 women, used the presence or absence of colour flow in sections of a mass thought morphologically indeterminate or malignant to predict whether or not the mass was truly malignant. If a mass was thought to be morphologically benign then the presence or absence of colour flow was disregarded. This technique improved the confidence level, specificity and positive predictive value of grey-scale sonography; specificity rose from 82 to 97% and the positive predictive value from 63 to 91%. The same study also confirmed the limited value of spectral Doppler indices.

Our experience with a cohort of patients in Leeds[36] concurs with the poor results obtainable from spectral Doppler indices, but also indicates that an experienced observer with access to all the ultrasound

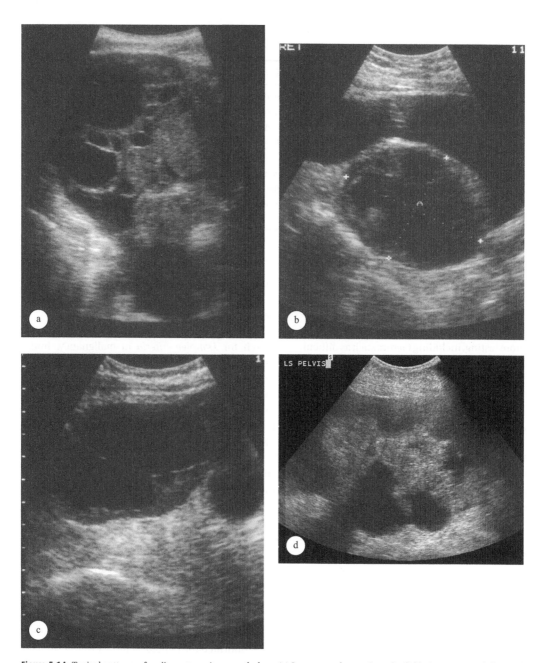

Figure 5.14 Typical patterns of malignant ovarian morphology. (a) Large complex cystic and solid lesion on transabdominal scanning in a 52-year-old woman. (b) Thick-walled cyst with internal nodules or papillae lying behind the bladder in a 56-year-old woman. (c) Relatively simple cyst with a fine septum but also with a small solid component in an 80-year-old woman. All these lesions were malignant. (d) A large ovarian malignancy showing the typical mixed solid and cystic morphology.

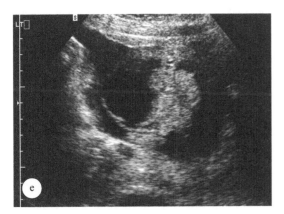
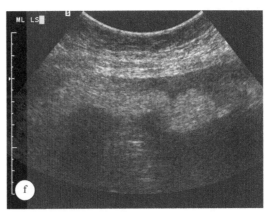

Figure 5.14 (*cont.*) (e) A smaller cyst showing an irregular mass arising out of one wall. There is free fluid. The mass is typical for malignancy. (f) Omental 'cake' surrounded by ascites. The ultrasound operator should always examine the rest of the abdomen when a suspected ovarian malignancy is found. Ultrasound is not sensitive to the presence of tumour spread but it is highly specific. Hence if tumour spread is found, then an advanced stage of malignant disease can be diagnosed.

information (i.e. morphology and Doppler indices) can outperform any of the individual scoring systems currently available. This multiparameter analysis by experienced observers is also now advocated by Kurjak and Kupesic,[37] who go on to describe the need for 'artistic rendering' in obtaining and interpreting results (Table 5.2).

Ultrasound contrast agents have been shown in two small studies to improve the diagnostic accuracy of power Doppler ultrasound in the diagnosis of early ovarian cancer.[38,39] These data need to be confirmed with larger-scale trials to ensure that this is not another false dawn in ovarian ultrasound imaging.

Metastases to ovary

Metastatic involvement of the ovaries from a distant primary tumour represents 10% of all ovarian malignancies. The primary tumour is sometimes only detected during investigation of the ovarian lesion. A Krukenberg tumour describes the spread of mucinous breast or gastrointestinal tract malignancy (from the colon, stomach and pancreas) to the ovaries. They may spread by direct invasion, intraperitoneal seeding, lymphatic or vascular routes. Tumours are most often bilateral solid lesions with a cystic component; bilaterality is

the first indicator to alert the sonographer that the ovaries may be involved in malignant disease from a distant site. This should then prompt a thorough

Table 5.2 Ultrasound features used in scoring systems to differentiate benign from malignant ovarian masses

Morphology	
Size	Larger masses more likely to be malignant
Wall thickness	Thick-walled masses score more highly for malignancy than those with thin walls
Composition	Complex, mainly fluid masses score more highly for malignancy than simple cysts
	Papillae and thickened septa score highly
Doppler	
Presence/absence	Non-vascular masses more likely to be benign
Distribution	Masses confined to the wall or with a regular pattern are more likely to be benign than masses with irregular vascular distribution throughout
Resistance	Low-resistance (high end-diastolic flow velocity) scores more highly for malignancy

review of the rest of the abdomen for a primary site of disease. Often a past history of malignancy is present, sometimes many years after the initial treatment, and particularly so in patients with breast cancer. In such cases CT scanning is advised to assess other sites of disease and biopsy is essential to confirm the source of the disease and to plan the most appropriate treatment. Lymphoma and leukaemia may also involve the ovaries, producing solid lesions, as a part of a more generalised disease process.[40]

Ovarian cancer screeening

The aim of ultrasound screening of the ovaries is to detect malignant disease without resulting in a large number of operations for conditions that eventually turn out to be benign. Early studies with transabdominal scanning on asymptomatic women achieved a poor rate of 67 operations for every ovarian cancer found. This can be improved by narrowing the cohort of women to be scanned, by selecting a higher-risk subgroup, or by using transvaginal scans and sequential testing with follow-up scans and CA125. A family history of ovarian cancer reduces the number of operations for benign disease for each cancer detected from around 1 in 50 to 1 in 12. Transvaginal scans in postmenopausal women also reduce this rate to around 1 in 10, although some operators, for example Kurjak and colleagues, appear to do much better than others. Using CA125 as the primary screening tool before ultrasound reduces the benign operation rate further, but also has the potential to miss up to 50% of early-stage tumours. It is apparent that an ill-conceived programme has a huge potential to cause harm without necessarily improving ovarian cancer survival.

Several major trials are currently under way to determine whether population screening is a viable and effective use of health care resources. The UK Collaborative Trial of Ovarian Cancer Screening Study (UKCTOCSS) aims to screen 200 000 postmenopausal women (with a combination of CA125, followed by transvaginal ultrasound where this is

elevated). The UK Familial Ovarian Cancer Screening Study (UKFOCSS) will follow up 5000 women with a strong family history of ovarian cancer. The results of these studies should be available in the near future.

Summary of main points: screening for ovarian cancer

- Lifetime risk is approximately 1 in 70 women
- Screening tools include bimanual palpation, genetic testing, CA125 levels and ultrasound
- Screening currently suffers from low sensitivity (cancers are missed) and low specificity (too many false-positive results) which cause unnecessary intervention and distress
- Sensitivity and specificity are improved when the screened population is restricted to high-risk women > 45 years or with a family history of ovarian or breast cancer
- False-positive results due to physiological masses are minimised by scanning in the early part of the cycle (days 1–8) or by selecting only postmenopausal women for the screening programme
- The role of ultrasound is enhanced by using transvaginal and colour Doppler techniques
- Although scoring systems have had some success, the best results are obtained using knowledgeable and experienced interpretation
- There is no evidence to support screening of the general population

Fallopian tube and adnexal pathology

Pelvic inflammatory disease

PID is an infective condition, usually caused by ascending lower genital tract infection by *Chlamydia*, gonorrhoea, commensal organisms or, rarely, from tuberculosis. Up to 10% of women are affected during their lives and the incidence may be rising. Risk factors for infection include previous episodes of sexually transmitted disease, multiple partners,

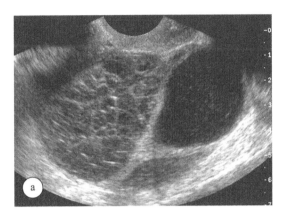

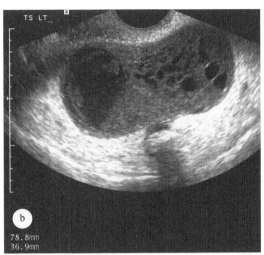

Figure 5.15   (a and b) Two examples of large complex tubo-ovarian abscesses.

presence of intrauterine contraceptive devices and septic abortion. A significant number of patients are presenting with infertility following an earlier asymptomatic infection or active chronic infection. In the acute setting patients complain of abdominal pain, dyspareunia, vaginal discharge and systemic upset, and often have raised inflammatory markers.

The inflammatory process has a range of ultrasound findings that reflects the distribution and severity of disease. In mild forms ultrasound is normal. Endometritis is essentially a clinical diagnosis but may be detected as endometrial thickening with fluid in the cavity and enlargement and hypoechogenicity of the myometrium.[41] However, the appreciation of mild enlargement can be difficult and endometrial thickening with fluid is a normal finding in the late stage of the cycle in reproductive-age women. As the fallopian tubes become involved they can become dilated, thick-walled and tortuous, containing fluid or echogenic blood or pus. Several descriptions have been allocated to the ultrasound appearances of the tubes, including the 'cogwheel sign' for the cross-sectional image of a dilated tube with thickened endosalpingeal walls and the 'string of beads sign' for mural nodules seen lining a dilated tube.[42] When the ovaries become caught up in the inflammatory process they may be seen closely applied to the uterus because of fibrosis and adhesions or, in the case of tubo-ovarian abscess, they may be no longer identified as separate from a complex inflammatory pelvic mass (Fig. 5.15). This mass can distort and obliterate all of the normal adnexal anatomy and image interpretation can be very difficult. Free fluid is often present but loculated collections or fluid-filled abscesses should be sought, as these can be successfully drained via transrectal or transvaginal routes using ultrasound guidance, thereby avoiding surgery to treat sepsis.[43,44] Pyosalpinx can also be treated effectively from drainage by this route.

Hydrosalpinx describes a dilated fluid-filled fallopian tube, arising from obstruction due to either previous PID or adhesions from surgery. They are either discovered incidentally or during imaging for causes of infertility. An apparently multiloculated mass adjacent to the ovaries may be seen or, more often, a fluid-filled tube with septations and kinking. Hystero-contrast sonography with Echovist (Shering, Germany) can assist in determining the anatomical structure of the blocked tube and allows assessment of tubal patency by demonstrating free flow of contrast into the pelvic peritoneal recesses.

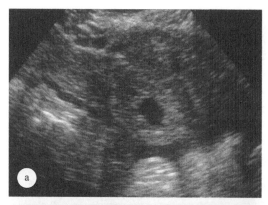

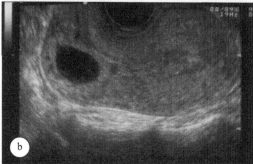

Figure 5.16 Ectopic pregnancy. (a) A typical adnexal ring structure is identified, together with surrounding echogenic free fluid. The echoes in the free fluid indicate the presence of a haemoperitoneum. The ring structure is the tubal pregnancy. (b) An example of a very rare cervical ectopic pregnancy. This can produce life-threatening haemorrhage.

Ectopic pregnancy

While this may present unexpectedly in a patient under investigation for infertility with an adnexal mass (Fig. 5.16), it more usually occurs in a patient with acute abdominal pain, vaginal bleeding and with a positive pregnancy test. The pregnancy test is the single most important investigation: a positive test makes the diagnosis highly likely. Serial serum beta-human chorionic gonadotrophic (β-HCG) measurements are a useful method of distinguishing early healthy pregnancy from ectopic pregnancy. In an ectopic pregnancy the normal doubling of β-HCG every 48 hours does not occur; an increase of less than 66% over 2 days is predictive of ectopic pregnancy. The imaging features and management of this condition are dealt with more fully in Chapter 6.

Broad-ligament fibroids

Occasionally uterine fibroids may extend into the broad ligament, simulating a solid adnexal mass. The diagnosis may be suggested by the presence of other uterine fibroids. Compression of adjacent structures can lead to fallopian tube and ureteric obstruction. Where there is doubt about the nature of the mass, MRI can be useful in further assessment. Fibroids are discussed more fully in Chapter 4.

Fallopian-tube carcinoma

This is a rare tumour, usually affecting postmenopausal women with a history of infertility. Patients present with bleeding, pain and, in some cases, with watery vaginal discharge. The ultrasound features are non-specific, but may include a cystic/solid adnexal mass in association with a unilaterally dilated fluid-filled tube. Clarification of the diagnosis may be possible with MRI before surgery. Standard surgical treatment is the same as for ovarian cancer, with hysterectomy, bilateral oophorectomy and omentectomy, as the tumour is bilateral in up to a quarter of patients and peritoneal dissemination is common.

Non-gynaecological pelvic pathology

Appendicitis

Appendicitis may produce non-specific symptoms in a significant number of patients, but most suffer abdominal pain with raised white cell count and inflammatory markers on blood-testing. The clinical picture in young women can mimic ectopic pregnancy, PID and torsion of the ovaries. In any female patient with abdominal pain the appendix may reasonably feature on the clinical differential diagnosis.

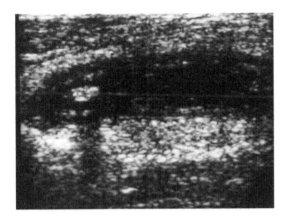

Figure 5.17 Appendicitis. There is a tubular, non-compressible structure containing an echogenic focus – an appendicolith. The walls of the appendix demonstrate the typical layered appearance seen in all bowel wall.

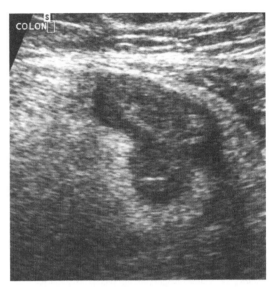

Figure 5.18 Diverticulitis. Note the bright inflamed mesenteric fat surrounding the outpouched diverticulum.

The imaging characteristics of the appendix when inflamed are of a blind-ending intestinal loop arising from the caecum, which is non-compressible, not peristalsing and measuring >6 mm in diameter (Fig. 5.17). A hyperechoic appendicolith may be present. Associated free fluid and increased echogenicity of the adjacent mesenteric fat may be present.

Bowel-related pathology

Diverticulitis is another common condition, which results in herniation of the colonic mucosa through its outer muscular wall. These outpouchings may become obstructed and inflamed, resulting in an episode of diverticulitis. The left colon is most commonly affected, particularly the sigmoid. Ultrasound of the bowel shows transmural thickening centred on a hypoechoic area (the diverticulum) protruding through the bowel wall. Once again, hyperechoic inflammatory change in adjacent mesenteric fat is a useful sign (Fig. 5.18). *Inflammatory bowel disease,* which incorporates Crohn's disease and ulcerative colitis, may be detected on ultrasonography as the cause of abdominal pain in some patients. A history of prior altered bowel habit, blood or mucus in stools or weight loss is typically present. There is wall-thickening with increased blood flow in active disease. The colon and distal small bowel may be inflamed in either condition but when fistulae and abscesses related to affected loops are present, a more specific diagnosis of Crohn's disease is suggested. *Colorectal cancer* may be demonstrated as a bowel-based soft-tissue mass with associated lymphadenopathy. Invasion of neighbouring viscera, such as the bladder, may be seen.

Renal tract and vascular pathology

A range of incidental abnormalities may be seen during pelvic ultrasound examination including *ureteric dilatation,* with accompanying *ureteric calculi* or *ureteroceles* and *bladder tumours* (Fig. 5.19). Sometimes it may not be clear from the history whether blood loss is per vaginam or per urethram. Bladder tumours are relatively common in the elderly population and the ultrasound operator needs to be alert to this possibility in someone presenting with

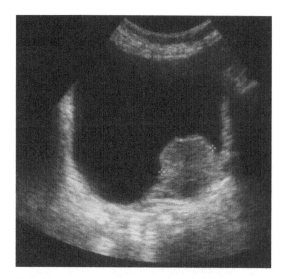

Figure 5.19 A large bladder tumour. Haematuria may be mistaken for postmenopausal bleeding by the patient, so be alert for alternative diagnoses during gynaecological scans.

supposed postmenopausal bleeding. *Iliac artery aneurysms* can also be discovered, often as an incidental finding, and sometimes are the explanation for pelvic pain symptoms. The use of colour Doppler should readily prevent an aneurysm being misdiagnosed as an ovarian cyst.

REFERENCES

1. T. Reynolds, M. C. Hill and L. M. Glassman, Sonography of hemorrhagic ovarian cysts. *Journal of Clinical Ultrasound*, **14** (1986), 449–53.

2. P. A. Athey and N. B. Cooper, Sonographic features of parovarian cysts. *American Journal of Roentgenology*, **144** (1985), 83–6.

3. M. B. Alpern, M. A. Sandler and B. L. Madrazo, Sonographic features of parovarian cysts and their complications. *American Journal of Roentgenology*, **143** (1984), 157–60.

4. Royal College of Obstetricians and Gynaecologists, Guideline no. 34. *Ovarian Cysts in Postmenopausal Women.* (London: Royal College of Obstetricians and Gynaecologists, 2003).

5. A. R. Nussbaum, R. C. Sanders, D. S. Hartman, D. L. Dugeon and T. H. Parmley, Neonatal ovarian cysts: sonographic-pathologic correlation. *Radiology*, **168** (1988), 817–21.

6. A. H. Balen, J. S. Laven, S. L. Tan and D. Dewailly, Ultrasound assessment of the polycystic ovary: international consensus definitions. *Human Reproduction Update*, **9** (2003), 505–14.

7. P. A. Athey and D. D. Diment, The spectrum of sonographic findings in Endometriomas. *Journal of Ultrasound Medicine*, **8** (1989), 487–91.

8. J. A. Spencer and M. J. Weston, Imaging in endometriosis. *Imaging*, **15** (2003), 63–71.

9. M. Bazot, R. Detchev, A. Cortez, *et al.*, Transvaginal sonography and rectal endoscopic sonography in the assessment of pelvic endometriosis: a preliminary comparison. *Human Reproduction*, **18** (2003), 1686–92.

10. R. Kumar, A. K. Haque and M. S. Cohen, Endometriosis of the urinary bladder: demonstration by sonography. *Journal of Clinical Ultrasound*, **12** (1984), 363–5.

11. G. Francica, C. Giardiello, G. Angelone, *et al.*, Abdominal wall endometriomas near cesarian delivery scars: sonographic and color Doppler findings in a series of 12 patients. *Journal of Ultrasound Medicine*, **22** (2003), 1041–7.

12. L. Fedele, S. Bianchi, A. Portese, F. Borruto and M. Dorta, Transrectal ultrasonography in the assessment of rectovaginal endometriosis. *Obstetrics and Gynecology*, **91** (1998), 444–8.

13. M. Graif and Y. Itzchak, Sonographic evaluation of ovarian torsion in childhood and adolescence. *American Journal of Roentgenology*, **150**, (1988), 647–9.

14. M. A. Warner, A. C. Fleisher, S. L. Edell, *et al.*, Uterine adnexal torsion: sonographic findings. *Radiology*, **154** (1985), 773–5.

15. C. L. Roberts and M. J. Weston, Bilateral massive ovarian edema: a case report. *Ultrasound in Obstetrics Gynecology*, **11** (1998), 65–7.

16. A. G. Shapiro, T. Thomas and M. Epstein, Management of hyperstimulation syndrome. *Fertility and Sterility*, **28** (1977), 237.

17. J. B. Rowlands, Hyper reactio luteinalis: a case report. *Journal of Clinical Ultrasound*, **6** (1978), 295.

18. H. E. Philips and J. P. McGahan, Ovarian remnant syndrome. *Radiology*, **142** (1982), 487–8.

19. B. Caspi, Z. Appelman, D. Rabinerson, *et al.*, Pathognomonic echo patterns of benign cystic teratomas of the ovary: classification, incidence and accuracy rate of sonographic diagnosis. *Ultrasound in Obstetrics and Gynecology*, **7** (1996), 275–9.

20. S. F. Quinn, Erickson and W. C. Black, Cystic ovarian teratomas: the sonographic appearance of the dermoid plug. *Radiology*, **155** (1985), 477–8.

21. W. M. Stephenson and F. C. Laing, Sonography of ovarian fibromas. *American Journal of Roentgenology*, **144** (1985); 1239–40.

22. E. K. Outwater, B. Marchetto and B. J. Wagner, Virilising tumours of the ovary: imaging features. *Ultrasound in Obstetrics Gynecology*, **15** (2000), 365–71.

23. P. A. Athey and R. S. Malone, Sonography of ovarian fibromas/thecomas. *Journal of Ultrasound in Medicine*, **6** (1987), 431–6.

24. J. Austoker, Screening for ovarian, prostatic, and testicular cancers. *British Medical Journal*, **309** (1994), 315–20.

25. NIH consensus development panel on ovarian cancer, Ovarian cancer: screening, treatment and follow up. *Journal of the American Medical Association*, **273** (1995), 491–7.

26. K. J. W. Taylor and P. E. Schwartz, Screening for early ovarian cancer. *Radiology*, **192** (1994), 1–10.

27. D. Ford, D. F. Easton and J. Peto, Estimates of the gene frequency of BRCAl and its contribution to breast and ovarian cancer. *American Journal of Human Genetics*, **57** (1995), 1457–62.

28. C. Lerman, S. Narod, K. Schulman *et al.*, BRCAl testing in families with hereditary breast–ovarian cancer. A prospective study of patient decision making and outcomes. *Journal of the American Medical Association*, **275** (1996), 1885–92.

29. A. Sassone, I. Timor-Tritsch, A. Artner, W. Carolyn and W. B. Warren, Transvaginal sonographic characterisation of disease: evaluation of a new scoring system to predict ovarian malignancy. *Obstetrics and Gynecology*, **78** (1991), 70–6.

30. S. Rottem, N. Levit, I. Thraler *et al.* Classification of ovarian lesions by high frequency transvaginal sonography. *Journal of Clinical Ultrasound*, **18** (1990), 359–63.

31. D. L. Brown, M. C. Frates, F. C. Laing *et al.*, Ovarian masses: can benign and malignant lesions be differentiated with color and pulsed Doppler US? *Radiology*, **190** (1994), 333–6.

32. L. Valentin, P. Sladkevicius and J. K. Marsa, Limited contribution of Doppler velocimetry to the differential diagnosis of extrauterine tumors. *Obstetrics and Gynecology*, **83** (1994), 425–33.

33. B. Bromley, H. Goodman and B. R. Benacerraf, Comparison between sonographic morphology and Doppler waveform for the diagnosis of ovarian malignancy. *Obstetrics and Gynecology*, **83** (1994), 434–7.

34. S. M. Stein, S. Laifer-Narin, M. B. Johnson *et al.*, Differentiation of benign and malignant adnexal masses: relative value of gray-scale, color Doppler, and spectral Doppler sonography. *American Journal of Roentgenology*, **164** (1995), 381–6.

35. J.-N. Buy, M. A. Ghossain, D. Hugol *et al.*, Characterization of adnexal masses: combination of color Doppler and conventional sonography compared with spectral Doppler analysis alone and conventional sonography alone. *American Journal of Roentgenology*, **166** (1996), 385–93.

36. L. I. G. Haigh, G. Lane and M. Weston, The role of Doppler ultrasound in the assessment of ovarian masses. *British Journal of Radiology*, **68**, (1995), 809.

37. A. Kurjak and S. Kupesic, Color Doppler imaging for the detection of ovarian malignancy is reliable (letter). *Ultrasound in Obstetrics and Gynecology*, **7** (1996), 380–3.

38. T. J. D'Arcy, V. Jayaram, M. Lynch *et al.*, Ovarian cancer detected non-invasively by contrast-enhanced power Doppler ultrasound. *British Journal of Obstetrics are Gynaecology*, **111** (2004), 619–22.

39. V. Sparac, S. Kupesic and A. Kurjak, What do contrast media add to three-dimensional power Doppler evaluation of adnexal masses? *Croatian Medical Journal*, **41** (2000), 257–61.

40. G. H. Bickers, J. J. Siebert, J. C. Anderson, S. Golladay and D. L. Berry, Sonography of ovarian involvement in childhood lymphocytic leukemia. *American Journal of Roentgenology*, **137** (1981), 399–401.

41. L. C. Swayne, M. B. Love and S. R. Karasick, Pelvic inflammatory disease: sonographic-pathologic correlation. *Radiology*, **151** (1984), 751–5.

42. I. E. Timor-Tritsch, J. P. Lerner, A. Monteagudo, K. E. Murphy and D. S. Heller, Transvaginal sonographic markers of tubal inflammatory disease. *Ultrasound in Obstetrics and Gynecology*, **12** (1998), 56–66.

43. J. L. Nosher, G. S. Needell, J. K. Amorosa and I. H. Krasna, Transrectal pelvic abscess drainage with sonographic guidance. *American Journal of Roentgenology*, **146** (1986), 1047–8.

44. J. L. Nosher, H. K. Winchman and G. S. Needell, Transvaginal pelvic abscess drainage with US guidance. *Radiology*, **165** (1987), 872–3.

6

Ultrasound in the acute pelvis

Hassan Massouh

Frimley Park Hospital, Frimley, Surrey

Introduction

Ultrasound is the first examination of choice in patients with acute pelvic pain, regardless of age, presentation or gender, and a more common request in females than males. Pelvic pain represents 10–15% of all urgent ultrasound examinations performed in a district general hospital (local audit) and results from a large variety of underlying causes, many of which may be gynaecological. The causes of pain vary and will depend upon the location, organ involved and underlying pathology such as infection, haemorrhage, infarct or ectopic pregnancy (EP).

The examination of choice in these circumstances is a combination of transabdominal (TA) and transvaginal (TV) ultrasound except in young girls and those with an intact hymen. The use of high-frequency vaginal probes and the proximity of the probe to the pelvic organs allow clear visualisation of the pelvic organs. The ability of the vaginal probe to touch the pelvic organs allows the sonographer to test for pain and detect the mobility of these organs, which are two important and useful signs in evaluating the cause of pelvic pain.

TA ultrasound is advantageous because of its ability to visualise large pelvic masses, detect the presence of ascites and examine other structures such as the kidneys and the other upper abdominal organs, which may be associated with the pain. However, TA ultrasound may be technically difficult in acute pelvic pain due to the presence of ileus, abdominal wall tenderness/rigidity and the lack of filling of the urinary bladder (which is frequently associated in particular with pelvic inflammation).

Prior to the ultrasound examination, the sonographer should obtain a full clinical history of the pain: its onset, frequency and relationship to menstrual cycle, its location, any associated fever, evidence of vaginal discharge, date of last menstrual period, past medical history and knowledge of previous surgery. This is essential information in helping the interpretation of the ultrasound findings.

Ectopic pregnancy

EP is defined as 'implantation of a fertilised ovum outside the uterine cavity'. Its incidence in the developed world is increasing[1,2] and it is associated with the use of intrauterine contraceptive devices, pelvic inflammatory disease, adhesions from previous EP and past pelvic surgery or corrective surgery for treating infertility (Table 6.1). Endometriosis, pelvic scarring and adhesions are also associated with an increased incidence of EP.

Patients with EP are usually women of child-bearing age, presenting with lower abdominal pain (more to the side of pregnancy) and tenderness, vaginal bleeding and history of missed or delayed period. It is possible for EP to pass undiagnosed in patients with minimal symptoms, in whom the implants die

Table 6.1 Factors associated with increased incidence of ectopic pregnancy

Use of contraceptive devices
Pelvic inflammatory disease
Previous pelvic surgery
Previous surgery for infertility
Endometriosis
Other causes of pelvic adhesions

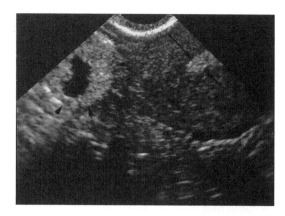

Figure 6.1 Transvaginal ultrasound showing right-sided ectopic pregnancy in the distal right tube (arrowheads) with decidual reaction of the endometrium (long arrows).

and the products resorb spontaneously. Confirming the presence of EP is usually by the history, clinical presentation, positive pregnancy test and positive hormone markers.

Ultrasound (particularly transvaginal) plays a major role in the early diagnosis of EP and its contribution to an accurate early diagnosis has reduced the mortality rate of EP. Over 95% of EP are within the fallopian tube (tubal) and the rest are intra-abdominal or intraperitoneal, ovarian, cervical or heterotopic.[3]

Ultrasound findings

The presence of a normal intrauterine pregnancy usually excludes EP except in very rare cases of heterotopic pregnancy, where there is an ectopic gestation with an intrauterine one.[3]

There is usually an adnexal or tubal mass consisting of an echogenic ring, representing the trophoblastic tissue, surrounding chorionic fluid. Depending on the age of the ectopic, it may be possible to see a yolk sac, fetal pole and also to detect a fetal heart beat, in which case the diagnosis is confirmed (Fig. 6.1). However, it is more common to find a complex mass on the side of the suspected EP and the contact of the vaginal probe with this mass is usually tender and painful. Care should be taken to differentiate between an ectopic sac and corpus luteal cyst, which is usually on the same side as the EP, by clearly identifying the ovary separately from the ectopic sac.

In the uterus, the endometrium is thickened as a result of decidual reaction, secondary to the effect of hormones. Fluid can accumulate with this decidual reaction, leading to what is described as

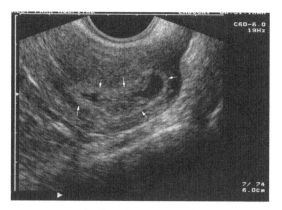

Figure 6.2 Transvaginal ultrasound of the uterus in a patient with an ectopic pregnancy showing fluid within the endometrial cavity with some thickening (decidual reaction) of the endometrium. Note the irregular margin of this fluid, which should not be mistaken for intrauterine pregnancy.

'pseudo-gestational sac' (Fig. 6.2). Compared with the true intrauterine sac, the pseudo-sac has an irregular margin, containing echogenic (bloody) fluid with absence of the 'double-ring border' of the normal intrauterine sac. Colour Doppler ultrasound can differentiate the hypervascular trophoblastic ring from the less vascular wall of the pseudo-sac. It is absolutely essential to examine both adnexae in all cases of an empty intrauterine sac in case it represents a pseudo-sac with an EP (Fig. 6.3).

Excess fluid in the pouch of Douglas, more than is usually present following ovulation, is also a positive sign of EP. The fluid may be bloody and echogenic (swirling motion of bloody fluid).

A pregnancy test is usually positive in both intra- and extrauterine gestation. The use of the discriminatory level of serum b human chorionic gonadotrophin (βhCG) has become widely used. It is now accepted that a normal intrauterine pregnancy should be detectable on transvaginal ultrasound if the serum βhCG is 1000 IU/l (second International Standard) or more. Failure to visualise intrauterine sac at this level of βhCG highly indicates either an EP or recent abortion.[4,5]

The value of serum progesterone for diagnosing EP remains equivocal, due to the overlap between normal and EP. Progesterone of ≥ 80 nmol/l indicates a normal intrauterine pregnancy in 98% of cases. Progesterone of < 16 nml/l indicates a non-viable pregnancy regardless of location. Most EPs will have a progesterone level of 32–60 nmol/l at presentation, significantly limiting the clinical usefulness of progesterone measurement in EP.[6]

It is important to remember that a negative ultrasound finding does not exclude EP. If there is clinical doubt about the diagnosis, follow-up scans and serial measurements are recommended.[7]

Ovarian and intra-abdominal EPs are rare and difficult to diagnose on ultrasound. They are usually found on laparoscopy following continuing clinical suspicion after a negative ultrasound.

Cervical pregnancy is also rare but can be diagnosed on TV ultrasound as a gestational sac in the cervical canal. It is a very painful type of EP and also dangerous, as it can bleed heavily.

Heterotopic pregnancy is very rare but its incidence is rising with the increasing use of reproductive or infertility procedures.[3] It consists of an intrauterine gestational sac in addition to an ectopic one (Fig. 6.4). It is good practice always to scan both adnexae during ultrasound in early pregnancy, particularly in those patients who have had fertility procedures.

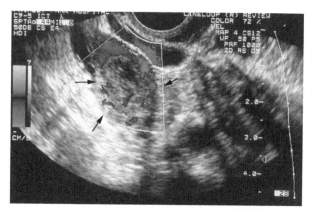

Figure 6.3 A young woman who had a dilatation and curettage for a suspected 7-week blighted ovum. The histological examination of the curetted tissue showed no fetal or trophoblastic tissue. Repeated transvaginal colour Doppler ultrasound showed right-sided ectopic pregnancy (arrowed). Note the increased vascularity of the trophoblastic tissue. What was thought to be a blighted ovum was, in retrospect, a pseudo-sac.

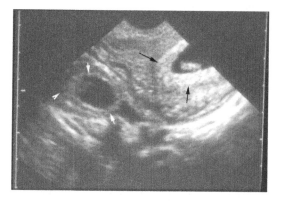

Figure 6.4 Heterotopic pregnancy: intrauterine gestational sac (long arrows) as well as a right-side ectopic pregnancy (arrowheads) in a 34-year-old woman who had fertility treatment using Clomid.

Surgery, whether open or laparoscopic, is usually the treatment for EP. However, non-surgical treatment is gathering popularity, particularly the use of methotrexate as a single dose.[8,9] Only selected patients meet the criteria for this type of treatment.

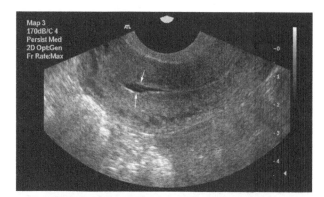

Figure 6.5 Fluid within the endometrial cavity (arrows) in a woman who developed acute endometritis and pelvic inflammatory disease following a difficult removal of an intrauterine contraceptive device.

Pelvic inflammatory disease

Pelvic inflammatory disease (PID) is the result of an infection by an organism spreading from the vagina to the fallopian tubes and ovaries via the endometrial cavity. The commonest organisms are *Chlamydia trachomatis* and *Neisseria gonorrhoeae*, although other organisms have been found to cause this infection, such as *Mycoplasma genitalium* and anaerobes.[10]

Various factors have been associated with the risk of developing PID, such as instrumentation of the cervix, abortion, hysteroscopy, contraceptive devices and other already existing pelvic infections such as appendicitis and diverticulitis.

PID markedly increases the risk of infertility, EP and chronic pelvic pain. UK national guidelines on sexually transmitted infection[11] were published in 2002, highlighting the increasing rate of gonorrhoea and the likelihood of increased risk of gonorrhoea PID in future. The Royal College of Obstetricians and Gynaecologists issued guidelines[12] stressing the need for good management of acute PID.

A further possible complication in patients with a history of PID is Fitz-Hugh and Curtis syndrome, an inflammation of the space around the liver capsule secondary to repeated *Chlamydia* infection.

The clinical symptoms on presentation of PID vary. In low-grade cases patients present with mild lower abdominal pain and tenderness. In moderate to severe cases, patients experience severe pelvic pain, fever, deep dyspareunia, cervical discharge, elevated white blood count, high C-reactive protein and erythrocyte sedimentation rate, although blood culture is rarely positive.

PID is primarily a clinical diagnosis. However, ultrasound, particularly TV ultrasound, remains the examination of choice in diagnosing any complication of PID.[13] Other imaging, such as magnetic resonance imaging (MRI) of the pelvis, has also been used for diagnosing PID.[14] Doppler ultrasound has been shown to be useful during TV ultrasound for the diagnosis of PID and inflammatory masses,[15,16] showing increased vascularity, hyperaemia and reduced level of pulsatility and resistance indices.

Ultrasound findings

Pain and tenderness are experienced during TV ultrasound when the probe is in contact with the cervix or the adnexae, reflecting the degree of underlying inflammation. This is the most common and possibly the only sign observed during TV ultrasound.

Fluid within the endometrial cavity in response to local endometritis is also seen, usually in small quantities (Figs. 6.5 and 6.6). This retained fluid may be echogenic or echo-poor, distending the endometrial cavity and outlining the surrounding endometrium. Vaginal discharge is commonly associated with the presence of retained fluid in the endometrial cavity.

Free fluid in the pelvis is a common finding and represents a reaction to pelvic inflammation.

Pure inflammation of the fallopian tube may not be confidently diagnosed on TV ultrasound unless the wall of the tube is thickened. Timor-Tritsch *et al.*[17] concluded that a tube wall of 5 mm or more determines pathological thickness. The wall thickness is seen along the length of the tube from cornua to ovary or on a transverse section through the thickened part of this tube. Retained infected fluid can be seen in the fallopian tube in acute cases, representing pyosalpinx. This appears as a tubal, oval-shaped

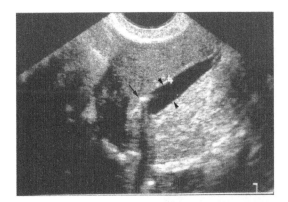

Figure 6.6 Transvaginal ultrasound in a 51-year-old woman with acute endometritis and pelvic inflammatory disease following hysteroscopy. Note the fluid within the endometrial cavity (arrowheads) and the small air bubble, presumably retained from the previous procedure (long arrow), which was observed to be mobile during scanning.

structure extending from the cornua to the ovary. The amount of fluid and distension of the tube's lumen vary. The wall of the tube becomes noticeably thickened and easily measurable and the fluid within the tube may be echogenic (see section on hydrosalpinx, below).

When the inflammation extends into the adnexal area, adhesions occur between the nearby structures, mainly the tube, ovary and bowel, leading to the formation of an inflammatory tubo-ovarian complex. In acute cases, this complex is referred to as a tubo-ovarian abscess because of the acute nature of the underlying infection (Fig. 6.7). Ultrasonically, this tubo-ovarian abscess appears as an ill-defined, relatively hypoechoic tender mass with a lack of anatomical differentiation of the normal structures of this part of the pelvis. A small collection of fluid may be seen within this mass or nearby, representing abscess formation.[17]

Chronic tubo-ovarian complex mass can also be caused by adhesions from previously treated PID and/or tubo-ovarian abscess. Although its ultrasonic appearance may be similar to the acute phase, there is usually less tenderness on TV ultrasound and less vascular hyperaemia. The history of previously treated PID, absence of inflammatory markers, plus the different clinical presentation at the time of

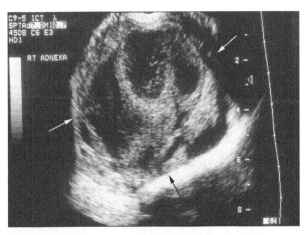

Figure 6.7 Tubo-ovarian abscess seen during a transabdominal ultrasound on a 28-year-old woman known to have had pelvic inflammatory disease, and who presented with right pelvic pain and signs of infection. Note the inflammatory complex mass (arrowed) consists of areas of increased reflectivity as well as pockets of echo-free fluid. Similar appearances can be seen in other causes of inflammation such as in Crohn's disease or following appendicitis.

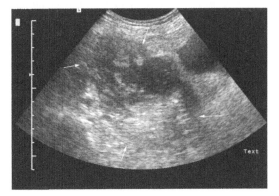

Figure 6.8 A 52-year-old woman with right pelvic pain. Transabdominal ultrasound showed a heterogeneous mass (arrowed) of mixed echogenicity which was mildly tender and was thought to be an adnexal inflammatory mass. At operation, it was found to be an inflammatory mass originating from an inflamed appendix.

attending for the ultrasound scan, usually help to confirm the chronic nature of this complex mass. Chronic inflammatory tubo-ovarian abscess can be similar to masses caused by other inflammation such as appendicitis or Crohn's disease (Fig. 6.8).

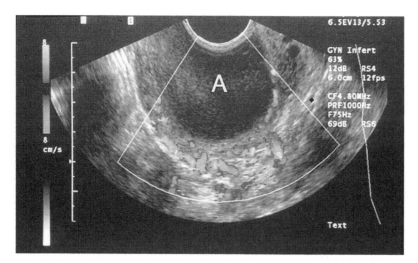

Figure 6.9 Transvaginal colour Doppler ultrasound of a young sexually active girl who was also known to have pelvic inflammatory disease. Note the fluid collection representing an abscess (A) near the vaginal vault and also the hypervascularity of the wall and nearby tissue, representing hyperaemia as a reaction to the inflammation.

Occasionally a large abscess may be seen in the adnexal area as a thick-walled fluid-filled cavity (Fig. 6.9). In this case the patient will have all the clinical signs and symptoms of the presence of an abscess.

Management of PID involves treatment with broad-spectrum antibiotics, either oral or intravenous, depending on the severity of the disease.[18] In case of the presence of pelvic abscess, TV ultrasound-guided drainage may be required.[19] Intrauterine devices must be removed in severe cases.

Hydrosalpinx

Hydrosalpinx is a Greek word, meaning fallopian tube filled with fluid. Although a normal tube is not usually visualised on routine TV ultrasound unless surrounded by adjacent fluid, it becomes noticeable and obvious when it is filled with fluid or when its wall becomes thickened. Hydrosalpinx is commonly the result of previous acute salpingitis and PID but has also been reported following pelvic surgery such as hysterectomy. It is usually unilateral but can also be bilateral. It is one of the common causes of infertility

and the presence of hydrosalpinx adversely affects the clinical pregnancy rate achieved with in vitro fertilisation[20] due to the direct toxic effect of the tubal fluid on the endometrium and the embryo.[21]

Pyosalpinx is when the fluid within this distended tube becomes infected. It is found either as part of acute PID or as an infection developed on an existing hydrosalpinx. The clinical symptoms of pyosalpinx are similar to acute PID. The fluid within the tube is usually echogenic (Fig. 6.10). Timor-Tritsch et al.[17] have described a 'Beads-on-a-string' sign which represents hyperechoic mural nodules arising from the wall of tube, projecting into the fluid-filled lumen and measuring 2–3 mm, indicating underlying inflammation. The appearance of the cross-section of the fluid-filled, inflamed, thickened tube has also been described by the same authors as 'cogwheel sign'.

Non-complicated hydrosalpinx is usually seen as an incidental finding and the fluid within it is usually echo-free (Fig. 6.11). It appears as a tortuous/coiled well-defined fluid-filled structure, oval-shaped and extending from the cornua to the ovaries. Its width varies from a few millimetres to a few centimetres depending on the amount of retained fluid within it.

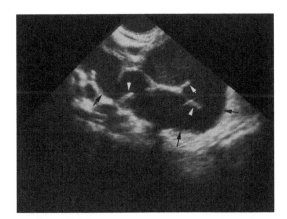

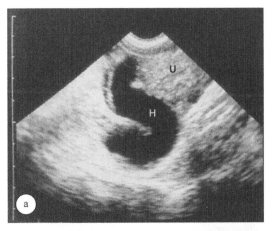

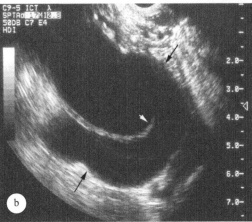

Figure 6.10 Transvaginal ultrasound of a young woman with acute pelvic pain and clinical picture of pelvic inflammation. Note the dilated tubular structure representing a hydrosalpinx (black arrows). Note that the fluid within the dilated tube is echogenic. White arrows are pointing to the folds which do not cross the entire lumen, as usually seen in septated ovarian cyst.

Often it is mistaken for a multicystic adnexal mass (Fig. 6.12) or septated ovarian cyst. The apparent septa, in reality the folded wall of the tube, do not cross the lumen completely (Figs. 6.10 and 6.11) and, by rotating the vaginal probe round in a fixed position, the operator will realise that all these 'apparent cysts' are communicating and part of one lumen. It is important to visualise the ovary on the same side as the tortuous hydrosalpinx, which is often mistaken for multiple large follicles.

Torsion of hydrosalpinx is a well-known complication, particularly when it is large, due to the weight of the fluid within it. The fluid becomes echogenic rather than echo-free, due to the underlying haemorrhage (see adnexal torsion below). A twisted hydrosalpinx can resemble ovarian torsion on ultrasound, making the definitive diagnosis difficult.

Other imaging modalities have been described and used in diagnosing hydrosalpinx such as MRI[22] and colour Doppler sonography. Guerriero *et al.*[23] have found that adding colour Doppler energy technique does not increase the diagnostic accuracy of TV ultrasound and found that TV ultrasound alone has a sensitivity and specificity of 84% and 99% respectively, with negative predictive value of 99%.

Figure 6.11 (a and b) Two examples of hydrosalpinx (H) seen on transvaginal ultrasound in two different women who had vague pelvic symptoms, which were probably unrelated to the findings. The folds (arrows) do not fully cross the lumen. U, uterus.

Haemorrhagic ovarian cyst

Haemorrhagic ovarian cyst (HOC) is usually seen in adults and premenopausal women, although it is also seen and reported in prepubertal children. It may also be seen in postmenopausal women who are on hormonal treatment.

Haemorrhagic corpus luteum is the commonest type of HOC, although haemorrhage into an existing cyst can also occur.

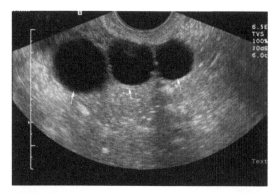

Figure 6.12 Transvaginal ultrasound, longitudinal section through a tortuous hydrosalpinx (arrows) resembling multiple adnexal cysts.

Table 6.2 Typical sonographic appearance of a haemorrhagic cyst throughout the staging process

Fine reticular pattern
Retracting blood clot
Fluid debris level
Haemorrhagic ovarian cyst simulating ectopic pregnancy
Haemorrhagic ovarian cyst simulating ovarian neoplasm
Haemorrhagic ovarian cyst simulating solid ovarian mass

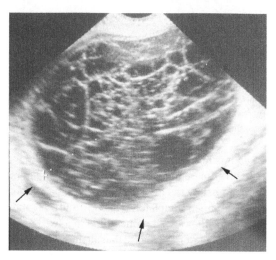

Figure 6.13 Transvaginal ultrasound of a young 24-year-old woman who presented with acute pelvic pain, showing an acute haemorrhage within a cyst proven at surgery. Note that the ultrasonic appearance can mimic a septated ovarian neoplasm.

Although HOC is sometimes seen in asymptomatic patients, it usually presents with sudden lower abdominal pain localised primarily to one side of the pelvis. Unless the level of the blood haemoglobin is low caused by the severe haemorrhage, all blood and biochemical tests are usually normal.

TV ultrasound in conjunction with the clinical history is the examination of choice for the diagnosis.[24,25] TV ultrasound is usually painful, particularly when touching the affected cyst. The appearance of the cyst and haemorrhage within it varies. In most cases, and unless the cyst has ruptured, a low-level echogenic mass is seen in the adnexal area and is inseparable from the ovary.

The appearance of the haemorrhage within the cyst depends on the timing of the scan in relation to the onset of pain. Kiran and Jain[26] have elegantly described all the typical sonographic appearances of the imaging spectrum listed in Table 6.2. During the acute stage, the cyst is full of echogenic material representing the echogenic blood (Fig. 6.13). Later on, a clot is formed and the cyst contains combined echogenic retracted clot next to echo-poor fluid (Fig. 6.14). At a much later stage, the clot retracts towards the wall of the cyst and appears like a filling defect within a fluid-filled structure or like a soft-tissue mass within a cyst (hence the importance not to call this a soft-tissue papillary projection into an ovarian cyst). Gentle compression of the cyst (during TV scanning with the patient lying on her side) confirms the mobility of this filling defect and identifies it as a blood clot. All these appearances relate to the different stages of the haemorrhage and the way it tends to evolve.

HOC can spontaneously rupture, leading to haemoperitoneum. In this case, an adnexal cyst may not be seen but echogenic fluid is observed in the peritoneal cavity, particularly in the pouch of Douglas. In this particular case, findings can mimic other causes of acute abdominal pain such as EP, ruptured ovarian torsion or PID.[27,28]

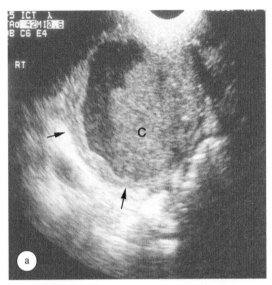

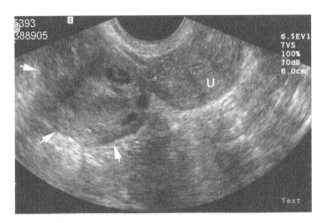

Figure 6.15 Ovarian torsion: 24-year-old woman with sudden severe right-sided pelvic pain. Transvaginal ultrasound showed torsion of the right ovary (arrows) next to the uterus (U).

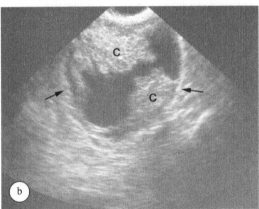

Figure 6.14 (a and b) Examples of haemorrhagic cysts (arrows). Note the retracted clots (C) within these cysts.

Adnexal torsion

Adnexal torsion is an acute medical condition where the ovary, ipsilateral fallopian tube or both rotate around its vascular pedicle, leading to vascular compromise.[29] It is commonly seen in young and middle-aged women but also reported in childhood and adolescents.[30,31] Adnexal torsion in elderly women is almost always associated with underlying adnexal mass.

Clinical presentation and symptoms can be misleading, making the diagnosis challenging and difficult. Symptoms vary according to the degree of twist (180–360°) and the underlying associated vascular insult. In mild rotation, lymphatic congestion is noted but both arterial and venous flow are present. Further torsion can compromise the venous return and more complete torsion will compromise the arterial blood supply and cause total necrosis of the ovary. Because the clinical symptoms are non-specific, presentation may resemble other causes of acute pelvic pain such as HOC, PID, EP and others. Therefore the diagnosis should be considered in the appropriate clinical picture. Often, ovarian torsion is associated with ipsilateral ovarian mass[29,32] and is more common on the right side than on the left,[33] probably due to the fact that the sigmoid colon occupies the left side of the pelvis.

The ultrasound findings vary but the commonest finding is an ovarian enlargement which is primarily due to lymphatic or lymphatic plus venous congestion of the ovary. Enlargement of the remaining follicle at the periphery of the ovary has been noted[30] (Fig. 6.15). The presence of an ovarian mass, whether it is cystic or solid, is common (Figs 6.16–6.18). Like other causes of acute pelvic pain, fluid in the pouch of Douglas is also a common finding and may be

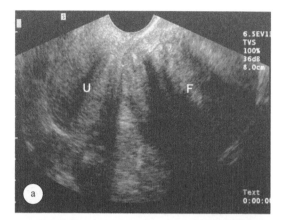

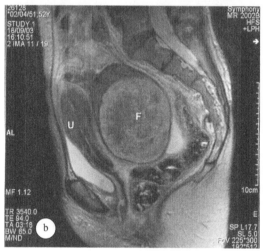

Figure 6.16 Twisted fibroma. (a) A 44-year-old woman collapsed with severe lower abdominal pain, which lasted for approximately 4 hours. Transvaginal ultrasound during the acute phase showed a large mass, which ultrasonically looks like a fibroid (F), separated from the uterus (U). (b) Magnetic resonance imaging scan of the pelvis demonstrated a mass-like fibroid (F), behind the uterus (U). At laparoscopy, a partially twisted broad-ligament fibroma was found. The patient was treated conservatively.

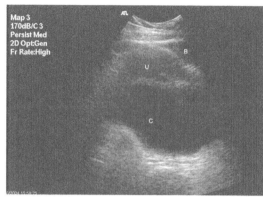

Figure 6.17 Twisted ovarian cyst: a 38-year-old Afro-Caribbean woman presented with severe lower abdominal pain. Transvaginal ultrasound was not useful. Transabdominal ultrasound demonstrated a large cystic mass (C) behind the uterus (U) which was displaced anteriorly behind the bladder (B). Laparotomy showed a large twisted ovarian cyst.

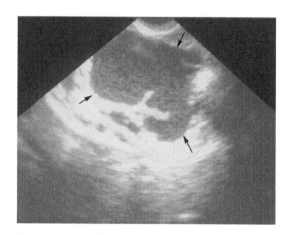

Figure 6.18 Twisted hydrosalpinx on transvaginal ultrasound on a middle-aged woman with severe lower abdominal pain. Transvaginal ultrasound demonstrated echogenic fluid within a hydrosalpinx (arrows). This was confirmed at laparotomy.

echo-free or echogenic in reflectivity. Compression of the torsed ovary by the transvaginal transducer is usually tender and triggers similar pain to that which the patient has been experiencing.

The use of colour Doppler as well as power Doppler has been described as a useful method for diagnosing torsed ovary.[33–35] Dilated vessels, particularly veins, are seen around the torsed ovary with absence of vessels within its substance. Colour Doppler ultrasound can visualise the pedicle of the torsed ovary and show the abrupt interruption of the arterial supply and venous drainage. However the presence of arterial and venous flow does not exclude the diagnosis of ovarian torsion.

Shalev *et al.*[35] have published 14 cases of what they described as subtorsion, which is a twist of the ovarian pedicle less than 360°. They found that torsed ovary may not be significantly enlarged, particularly if compared with the normal side, and that blood flow, both arterial and venous, can be still detected in the ovary. Congested and dilated periovarian vessels were also a common finding. They also found that fluid in the pouch of Douglas is not common in the subtorsion type.

Although sonography, particularly TV ultrasound with colour Doppler, is usually the most readily available and used modality for diagnosing torsion, other imaging techniques like CT and MRI have been used for this diagnosis and play a role, particularly in the subacute cases.[36]

The active diagnosis of this condition is very important, particularly as early diagnosis and surgical treatment can save the ovary from developing irreversible ischaemia and necrosis.

Non-gynaecological pelvic inflammation

Appendicitis

Appendicitis is a common cause of right iliac fossa pain, frequently occurring in children and adolescents but also seen in patients of any age. Diagnosis is usually made on clinical grounds based on the presenting symptoms in conjunction with the elevated white blood cell count and inflammatory markers. In most cases, the entire appendix is usually inflamed and all layers are affected and thickened (Fig. 6.19). However, inflammation of part of the appendix, usually the tip, can also occur.[37] The underlying inflammation may lead to local perforation and the formation of an abscess or inflammatory complex mass.

Imaging is commonly used, particularly in young females, to exclude any other cause of the pain such as ovarian/adnexal. Ultrasound is the most readily available and commonly used modality for diagnosing this condition. Ultrasonic visualisation

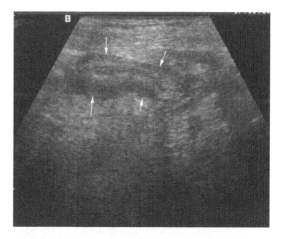

Figure 6.19 Acute appendicitis in a middle-aged woman: the appendix has a sausage shape, and is non-compressible with thickening of all layers (arrows).

of the inflamed appendix or the inflammatory mass is often hampered by the presence of local ileus and dilated loop of bowel and also by the local pain and abdominal wall rigidity.

Graded compression technique[38] has been described as a useful method of visualising the inflamed appendix which involves scanning at a different degree of compression over the site of appendix.

The transverse section of the normal appendix appears either rounded or ovoid. Rettenbacher *et al.*,[39] in a large prospective study, showed that a rounded appendix raises the suspicion of an underlying inflammation but only with specificity and positive predictive value of 37% and 50% respectively. They also concluded that an ovoid-shape transverse section over the entire appendiceal length reliably rules out acute appendix.

Poortman *et al.*[40] found that an incompressible appendix with a transverse diameter of 6 mm or more, with and without appendicolith, indicated appendicitis. The inflamed appendix appears as a blind-ended sausage shape on longitudinal scan (Fig. 6.19). Appendicolith may be seen within its lumen as a hyperreflective structure (Fig. 6.20a). The inflamed appendix may be part of an inflammatory

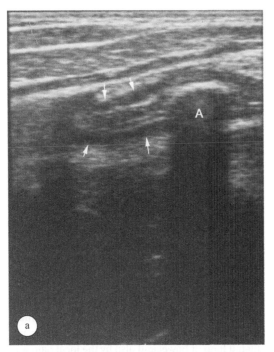

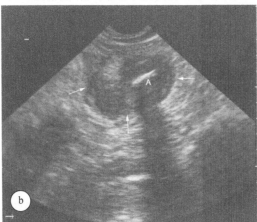

Figure 6.20 Acute appendicitis. (a) Transabdominal ultrasound using a high-frequency linear transducer: sausage-shape inflamed appendix (arrows) with appendicolith (A) at its base. (b) Inflammatory appendicular mass: transvaginal ultrasound on a patient with clinical signs of appendicitis showed a relatively hypoechoic inflammatory mass (long arrows) surrounding an inflamed appendix with appendicolith (A) within it, proven at surgery.

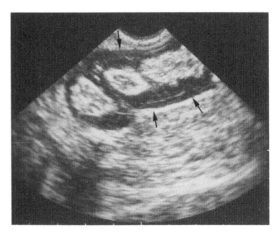

Figure 6.21 Crohn's colitis: transvaginal ultrasound on a 24-year-old female with severe lower abdominal pain and diarrhoea showing thickening of the wall and mucosa of the pelvic colon (arrows). Colonoscopic-guided biopsy confirmed the diagnosis of Crohn's. Ulcerative colitis can give similar appearances.

mass or an abscess (Fig. 6.20b). In such a case, and without the presence of an appendicolith, the ultrasonic appearance may be similar to other causes such as PID and endometriosis. Fujii *et al.*,[41] in a large prospective study, found that the use of ultrasound in patients with suspected appendicitis increases the accuracy of the diagnosis, reduces unnecessary operations and provides more appropriate selection of patients' treatment.

Colitis

This is an inflammation of the bowel occurring in young patients, commonly in the form of ulcerative colitis and Crohn's disease. Ulcerative colitis exclusively affects the colon and Crohn's affects both small and large bowel. When the colon is affected, its wall becomes oedematous and thickened with thickening of the mucosa. The ultrasonic appearance reflects exactly these histological changes, showing thickened echo-poor muscularis and echogenic mucosa[42] (Fig. 6.21). Local abscesses

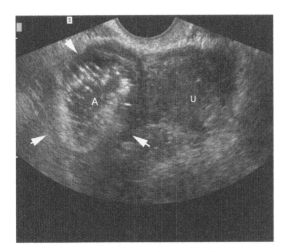

Figure 6.22 Crohn's abscess: transvaginal ultrasound on a female patient known to have Crohn's disease, demonstrating a fluid-filled abscess (A) to the right of and inseparable from the uterus (U) with high reflective speckles within it representing air bubbles.

are commonly seen more in Crohn's than in ulcerative colitis (Fig. 6.22).

Diverticulitis

This is an acute inflammation of the colon on an existing diverticular disease, usually affecting older people over the age of 50 and commonly affecting the sigmoid colon, causing thickening of the colonic wall and leading to narrowing of the lumen. This narrowing can sometimes be severe enough to cause sigmoid obstruction. Acute diverticulitis is commonly associated with pericolonic inflammation and adhesions and sometimes pericolic abscess.

It may be difficult to visualise any abnormality on pelvic ultrasound due to the ileus, abdominal pain and guarding. Usually, in the left lower part of the abdomen, a thick-walled sigmoid colon is seen with air passing within it (Fig. 6.23b) associated with focal tenderness when applying local pressure.[43] A local adjacent collection of echogenic fluid (pus) is often seen (Figs. 6.23a and 6.24). The position of pain, age of the patient and clinical history should be sufficient

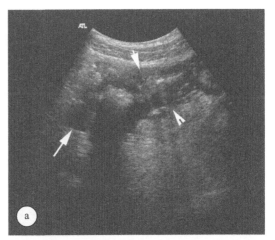

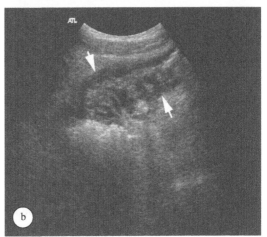

Figure 6.23 (a and b) Examples of acute diverticulitis on transvaginal ultrasound: note the thickening of the colonic wall (arrowheads) and the small nearby fluid collection representing an abscess (long arrow).

to differentiate this condition from other colitis such as Crohn's and ulcerative types.

Other causes of acute pelvic pain

Pelvic haemorrhage

Spontaneous pelvic haemorrhage is rare and usually occurs in patients on anticoagulation treatment. It

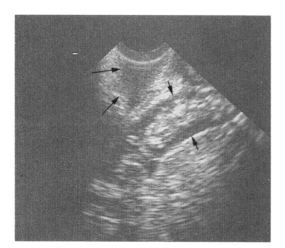

Figure 6.24 Acute diverticulitis with pericolic abscess: transvaginal ultrasound on an elderly lady showing thickened pelvic colon wall (short arrows) plus a nearby fluid collection/pus (long arrows) close to the vaginal vault.

is commonly localised to the abdominal wall more than the intraperitoneal space.

Postoperative haemorrhage/haematoma is a common complication. The haematoma is usually localised to the site of surgery and develops within the first few days following the operation. Post-hysterectomy (TA or TV) haematoma is common following gynaecological surgery. The haematoma is situated in the uterine bed or near the vaginal vault.

Ultrasonically, haematomas are hypoechoic, have ill-defined margins in the acute phase and can become localised and liquefied with time (Fig. 6.25). Colour Doppler scanning shows no vessels within it and this helps to differentiate haematomas from other echo-poor tumours such as lymphomas where vessels are seen within the tissue.

Haemorrhage within an ovarian cyst is already covered above. However, haemorrhage within a fibroid is rare but well-known. It occurs during pregnancy as a reaction of the fibroid to the maternal hormone (Fig. 6.26).

Endometriosis

This is covered more fully in Chapter 4 but is a well-known cause of acute pelvic pain. In most cases, the

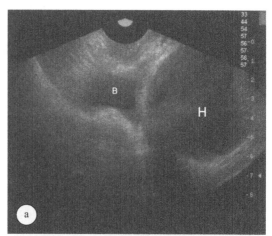

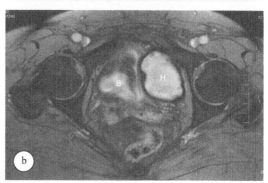

Figure 6.25 (a) Transvaginal ultrasound on a 64-year-old woman who developed urinary frequency and dysuria following pelvic surgery showing a large non-vascular echo-poor mass (H) in the left side of the pelvis classical of a haematoma. Note the displacement of the bladder (B). (b) T2-weighted spin-echo axial magnetic resonance imaging scan of the pelvis on the same patient 5 weeks after surgery showed the haematoma (H) as a high-signal mass due to the liquefication displacing the bladder (B).

patient gives a clear history of the disease and TV ultrasound is commonly the examination of choice in helping with the diagnosis (Fig. 6.27).

Imperforated hymen

This is a cause of an acute on chronic pelvic pain due to retention of the menstrual blood within the vagina.[44] TA ultrasound often demonstrates a fluid

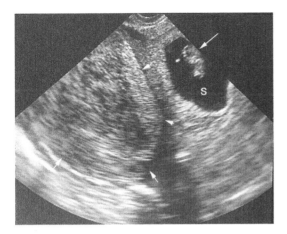

Figure 6.26 Haemorrhage within a fibroid: a 9-week pregnant woman presented to casualty with sudden severe lower pelvic pain. Previous pelvic ultrasound, before the pregnancy, had already identified a 4-cm uterine fibroid. Transvaginal ultrasound showed a viable fetus (long arrow) in a normally positioned gestational sac (S) with adjacent mass of mixed echogenicity representing haemorrhage within the fibroid (arrowed). This was proven at laparoscopy. The patient later miscarried.

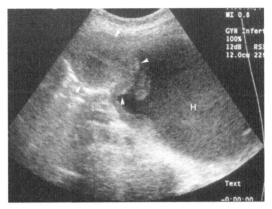

Figure 6.28 Imperforate hymen: a 14-year-old girl presented with lower abdominal pain which, on careful questioning, she had had intermittently for over a year. She had not had a period before. Transvaginal ultrasound showed the uterus displaced cranially by a large amount of echogenic fluid in the region of the vagina representing haematocolpos (H). On examination she was found to have an intact hymen.

collection in the region of the vagina with the uterus displaced cranially (Fig. 6.28). See also Chapter 8.

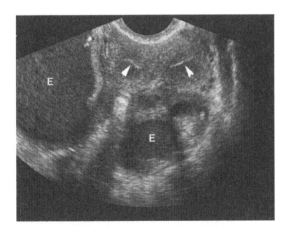

Figure 6.27 Endometriosis: transvaginal ultrasound on a female with a known history of endometriosis. Note the bicornuate uterus (arrowheads). The endometriotic cysts (E) are seen containing echogenic fluid (chocolate cysts). Note the lack of separation and tissue planes between the uterus and the surrounding structures due to adhesions.

REFERENCES

1. F. E. Skjeldestad, J. S. Kendrick, H. K. Atrash and A. K. Daltveit, Increasing incidence of ectopic pregnancy in one Norwegian county – a population based study, 1970–1983. *Acta Obstetrica Gynecologica Scandinavica*, **76** (1997), 159–65.

2. W. H. Chow, J. R. Daling, W. Cates *et al.*, Epidemiology of ectopic pregnancy. *Epidemiological Review*, **9** (1987), 71–94.

3. S. Ikeda, M. Sumiyoshi, M. Nakae *et al.*, Heterotopic pregnancy after in vitro fertilization and embryo transfer. *Acta Obstetrica Gynecologica Scandinavica*, **77** (1998), 463–4.

4. T. S. Mehta, D. Levine and B. Beekwith, Treatment of ectopic pregnancy: is a hCG level of 2000 mLU/ml a reasonable threshold? *Radiology*, **205** (1997), 569–73.

5. N. Kadar, M. Bohrer, E. Kemmann *et al.*, The discriminatory chorionic gonadotropin zone for endovaginal sonography: a prospective randomised study. *Fertility and Sterility*, **61** (1994), 1016–20.

6. R. Dart, P. Ramanujam and L. Dart, Progesterone as a predictor of ectopic pregnancy when the ultrasound is

indeterminate. *American Journal of Emergency Medicine*, **20** (2002), 575–9.

7. M. C. Frate and F. C. Laing, Sonographic evaluation of ectopic pregnancy: an update. *American Journal of Roentgenology*, **165** (1995), 251–9.

8. T. G. Stoval and F. W. Ling, Single dose methotrexate: an expanded clinical trial. *American Journal of Obstetrics and Gynecology*, **168** (1993), 1759–65.

9. M. Yao and T. Tulandi, Current status of surgical and nonsurgical management of ectopic pregnancy. *Fertility and Sterility*, **67** (1997), 421–33.

10. C. R. Cohen, L. E. Manhart, E. A. Bukusi *et al.*, Association between *Mycoplasma genitalium* and acute endometritis. *Lancet*, **359** (2002), 765–6.

11. Clinical Effectiveness Group, *UK National Guidelines on Sexually Transmitted Infections. 2002. Pelvic Inflammatory Disease*. Available online at: www.agum.org.uk/ceg2002/pid0601.htm.2002.

12. Royal College of Obstetricians and Gynaecologists, *Guidelines no. 32*. Acute Pelvic Inflammatory Disease, Management of (London: Royal College of Obstetricians and Gynaecologists, 2003).

13. D. I. Bulas, P. A. Ahlstrom, C. J. Sivit *et al.*, Pelvic inflammatory disease in the adolescent: comparison of transabdominal and transvaginal sonographic evaluation. *Radiology*, **183** (1992), 435–9.

14. T. A. Tukeva, H. J. Aronen, P. T. Karjalainen *et al.*, MR imaging in pelvic inflammatory disease: comparison with laparoscopy and US. *Radiology*, **210** (1999), 209–16.

15. H. Tikanen and E. Kujansuu, Doppler ultrasound findings in tubo-ovarian infectious complex. *Journal of Clinical Ultrasound*, **21** (1993), 175–8.

16. P. Molander, J. Sjoberg, J. Paavonen and B. Cacciatore, Transvaginal power Doppler findings in laparoscopically proven acute pelvic inflammatory disease. *Ultrasound in Obstetrics and Gynecology*, **17** (2002), 233–8.

17. I. E. Timor-Tritsch, J. P. Lerner, A. Monteagudo *et al.*, Transvaginal sonographic markers of tubal inflammatory disease. *Ultrasound in Obstetrics and Gynecology*, **12** (1998), 56–66.

18. J. D. C. Ross, Pelvic inflammatory disease: how should it be managed? *Current Opinion in Infectious Diseases*, **16** (2003), 37–41.

19. E. Van Sonnenberg, H. B. D'Agostino, G. Casola *et al.*, US-guided transvaginal drainage of pelvic abscesses and fluid collections. *Radiology*, **181** (1991), 53–6.

20. W. De Wit, C. J. Gowrising, D. J. Kuik *et al.*, Only hydrosalpinges visible on ultrasound are associated with reduced implantation and pregnancy rate after IVF. *Human Reproduction*, **13** (1998), 1696–701.

21. T. Mukherjee, A. B. Copperman, C. McCaffrey *et al.*, Hydrosalpinx fluid has embryotoxic effect on murine embryogenesis: a case for prophylactic salpingectomy. *Fertility and Sterility*, **66** (1996), 851–3.

22. E. K. Outwater, E. S. Siegelman, P. Chiowanich *et al.*, Dilated fallopian tubes: MRI imaging characteristics. *Radiology*, **208** (1998), 463–9.

23. S. Guerriero, S. Ajossa, M. P. Lai *et al.*, Transvaginal ultrasonography associated with colour Doppler energy in the diagnosis of hydrosalpinx. *Human Reproduction*, **15** (2000), 1568–72.

24. T. Okai, K. Kobayashi, E. Ryo *et al.*, Transvaginal sonographic appearance of hemorrhagic functional ovarian cyst and their spontaneous regression. *International Journal of Gynaecology and Obstetrics*, **44** (1994), 47–52.

25. O. H. Baltarowich, A. B. Kurtz, M. E. Pasto *et al.*, The spectrum of sonographic findings in hemorrhagic ovarian cyst. *American Journal of Roentgenology*, **148** (1987), 901–5.

26. A. Kiran and M. D. Jain, Sonographic spectrum of hemorrhagic ovarian cyst. *Journal of Ultrasound Medicine*, **21** (2002), 879–86.

27. J. G. Hallatt, C. H. Steele and M. Snyder, Ruptured corpus luteum with hemoperitoneum: a study of 173 surgical cases. *American Journal of Obstetrics and Gynecology*, **149** (1984), 5–9.

28. B. S. Hertzberg, M. A. Kliewer and E. K. Paaulson, Ovarian cyst rupture causing hemoperitoneum: imaging features and the potential for misdiagnosis. *Abdominal Imaging*, **24** (1999), 304–8.

29. L. T. Hibbard, Adnexal torsion. *American Journal of Obstetrics and Gynecology*, **152** (1985), 456–61.

30. M. Graif and Y. Itzchak, Sonographic evaluation of ovarian torsion in childhood and adolescence. *American Journal of Roentgenology*, **150** (1988), 647–9.

31. J. E. Stark and M. J. Siegel, Ovarian torsion in prepubertal and pubertal girls: sonographic findings. *American Journal of Roentgenology*, **163** (1994), 1479–82.

32. M. A. Warner, A. C. Fleischer, S. L. Edell *et al.*, Uterine adnexal torsion: sonographic findings. *Radiology*, **154** (1985), 773–5.

33. F. Albayram and U. M. Hamper, Ovarian and adnexal torsion: spectrum of sonographic findings with pathologic correlation. *Journal of Ultrasound Medicine*, **20** (2001), 1083–9.

34. E. J. Lee, H. C. Kwon, H. J. Joo *et al.*, Diagnosis of ovarian torsion with color Doppler sonography: depiction of twisted vascular pedicle. *Journal of Ultrasound Medicine*, **17** (1998), 83–9.

35. J. Shalev, R. Mashiach, I. Bar-Hava *et al.*, Subtorsion of the ovary: sonographic features and clinical management. *Journal of Ultrasound Medicine*, **20** (2001), 849–54.

36. S. E. Rha, J. Y. Byun, S. E. Jung *et al.*, CT and MR imaging features of adnexal torsion. *Radiographics*, **22** (2002), 283–94.

37. H. V. Nghiem and R. B. Jeffry, Jr., Acute appendicitis confined to the appendiceal tip: evaluation with graded compression sonography. *Journal of Ultrasound Medicine*, **11** (1992), 205–7.

38. J. B. C. M. Puylaert, Acute appendicitis: US evaluation using graded compression. *Radiology*, **158** (1986), 355–60.

39. T. Rettenbacher, A. Hollerweger, P. Macheiner *et al.*, Ovoid shape of the vermiform appendix: a criterion to exclude acute appendicitis – evaluation with US. *Radiology*, **226** (2003), 95–100.

40. P. Poortman, P. N. M. Lohle, C. M. C. Schoemaker *et al.*, Comparison of CT and sonography in the diagnosis of acute appendicitis: a blind prospective study. *American Journal of Roentgenology*, **181** (2003), 1355–9.

41. Y. Fujii, J. Hata, K. Futagami *et al.*, Ultrasonography improves diagnostic accuracy of acute appendicitis and provide cost saving to hospitals in Japan. *Journal of Ultrasound Medicine*, **19** (2000), 409–14.

42. M. E. O'Malley and S. R. Wilson, US of gastrointestinal tract abnormalities with CT correlation. *Radiographics*, **23** (2003), 59–72.

43. S. G. Parulekar, Sonography of colonic diverticulitis. *Journal of Ultrasound in Medicine*, **12** (1985), 659–66.

44. M. R. Spevak and H. L. Cohen, Ultrasonography of the adolescent female pelvis. *Ultrasound Quarterly*, **18** (2002), 275–88.

7

Ultrasound and fertility

Stephen Killick

Women and Children's Hospital, Hull

Introduction

Ultrasound is the single most useful agent in evaluating human fertility. Not only do the fluid–tissue interfaces in the female pelvic organs allow precise measurements of structure but the low cost and safety of ultrasound scanning allow repeated examinations and hence, most importantly, an understanding of function (Table 7.1).

Although transabdominal ultrasound is used occasionally, for example when surgery has moved ovaries from their normal location, the vast majority of scans are performed vaginally. The close proximity of the ovaries and uterus to the vaginal fornices allows for the use of higher frequencies (∼10 MHz) and hence higher resolution.

Subfertility is common. Some 19% of pregnancies take more than a year to conceive[1] and one in six of all couples are referred for fertility investigations at some time during their lives.[2]

Ovarian function

A human ovary contains many thousands of germ cells distributed throughout its stroma, each of which is surrounded by a small number of specialist cells to create a primordial follicle. These follicle complexes begin to develop one by one throughout reproductive life in response to gonadotrophin hormones secreted by the pituitary gland but they only become visible to ultrasound in their later stages of development when they develop a fluid-filled antrum. These fluid-filled follicles give the ovary its characteristic appearance during the reproductive years. When visualising the ovary it is important to remember that its structure is constantly changing as part of a dynamic system involving many other organs.

During an ovulatory cycle antral follicles increase in diameter by up to 2 mm a day in response to follicle-secreting hormone (FSH) secreted by the pituitary gland. The first follicle to begin development in any one month is the largest and is termed the first-order (graafian) follicle, with second- and third-order follicles following on behind. At mid-cycle the pituitary releases a surge of gonadotrophins (FSH and especially luteinising hormone (LH)) and the first-order follicle (and sometimes the second-order follicle as well) ovulates. Follicles are usually between 18 and 22 mm diameter when they ovulate but this is variable and they can be smaller or larger. Lower-order follicles are not mature enough to respond and slowly resolve. The release of follicular fluid at the time of ovulation can be seen by ultrasound to take several hours; it is not a sudden burst. The follicle shrinks to at least half its previous size and then grows into a corpus luteum, which is irregularly cystic and up to 3 cm in diameter. Whereas the first half of the ovarian cycle before ovulation can be of

Table 7.1 Advantages and disadvantages of ultrasound in evaluating fertility

Advantages	Disadvantages
Precise measurements of pelvic structures	Initial cost of machinery
Instant result	Operator-dependent
Viewed by the woman herself	Vaginal scan is personally invasive
Allows for simultaneous counselling	
Safe	
Inexpensive repeat measurements	
Used for oocyte capture	
Gives idea of function, not just structure	
Permanent record can be retained	

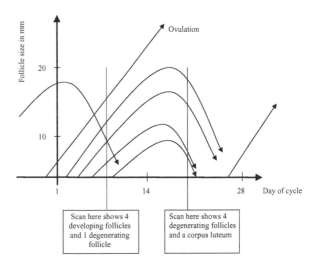

Figure 7.1 A schematic representation of how follicles develop and degenerate in the normal ovulating ovary, thus altering its ultrasound appearance.

variable duration, menstruation takes place 14 days after ovulation if conception does not occur.

A single view of a normal functioning ovary may, therefore, demonstrate a complex picture of several small newly developing follicles, some old degenerating follicles and a corpus luteum, all embedded in a solid vascular stroma. More useful information is gained by observing how the picture changes day by day (Fig. 7.1).

Premenarchal ovaries often contain antral follicles; in fact the ovaries of adolescent girls have multiple follicles, indicating that there is enough FSH to induce follicular growth but the pituitary has yet to mature and develop its feedback mechanism with the ovary in order to induce ovulation. This picture is also seen in other situations where pituitary function is compromised, such as weight-related amenorrhoea or anorexia nervosa. It can be confused with polycystic ovaries (PCO; see below) but in PCO there is an increased amount of ovarian stroma.

Towards the end of reproductive life as the menopause encroaches, multiple ovulations become more common, as does anovulation, and so the ovary may contain several quite large follicles. For this reason non-identical twins are more common in older women.

The endometrial cycle

The routine growth and shedding of the endometrial lining can also be monitored with ultrasound. During menstruation the endometrium appears somewhat irregular and highly reflective. The endometrium increases in thickness to about 1 cm in the first half of the cycle. At this stage, just prior to ovulation, it is of a lower echo intensity than the myometrium and is surrounded by a narrower layer of even lower echo intensity, the junctional zone. The junctional zone represents the innermost cells of the myometrium, which are more tightly packed than in the outer layer. After ovulation, under the influence of the hormone progesterone, the endometrial layer becomes more echo-intense than the myometrium (Fig. 7.2).

The ultrasonographer needs to remember functional interrelationships. Antral follicles secrete almost all of the body's oestrogen and so, for example, if an ovary is seen to contain a 2-cm-diameter echo-free cystic structure, then the woman is probably mid-cycle and the uterine endometrium will be several millimetres thick but still of low echo intensity. If this is not the case and the endometrium is

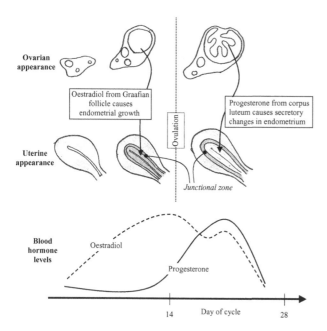

Figure 7.2 Diagram to illustrate the interrelationships between blood hormone levels and ovarian and uterine appearances throughout the ovulatory cycle.

thin (~4 mm) the cystic structure is not a graafian follicle producing oestrogen.

Management of subfertility

Subfertile couples need to be managed with sympathy. Information counselling and support counselling do not necessarily mean the intervention of a trained counsellor. An ultrasonographer is in an ideal situation to provide information and support whilst viewing the screen with the subfertile couple. To maximise this advantage the ultrasonographer must be part of the fertility team and should be aware of the clinical situation of each specific couple.

Each subfertile couple needs to have an estimate of their chances of natural conception before they decide whether to opt for treatment. In practice this needs a minimum of three assessments: an analysis of the male partner's ejaculate, an assessment of ovulation and some test of fallopian tube patency.

Ultrasound could be used for the diagnosis of ovulation but usually a more convenient way is to take a single blood sample for progesterone 7 days before the first day of the next period, when the value should be at its peak and greater than 30 nmol/l.

Tubal patency testing

Fallopian-tube patency can be visualised ultrasonographically if a positive contrast medium is used. The procedure is termed hystero-contrast sonography, or HyCoSy for short, and is recommended by the National Institute for Clinical Excellence (NICE) as the procedure of choice for initial determination of tubal patency.[3] A catheter is introduced through the cervix and held in place by inflating a small balloon at its tip. The commercially available material Echovist (Schering, UK) is then injected in volumes of less than 1 ml at a time whilst a vaginal scan is performed.[4]

Procedures are usually performed in the first half of the menstrual cycle, preferably before the endometrium has attained its maximum thickness and before any chance of pregnancy, although good results can be obtained at any stage of the cycle. Considerable experience of vaginal scanning is necessary for consistent results. The use of Doppler does not help in the assessment. HyCoSy may be combined with an initial assessment of the uterine cavity to exclude such things as uterine polyps, submucous fibroids or septa. In this case a negative contrast is much better and saline is usually used before any positive contrast is injected. This procedure is termed saline infusion sonography.

It has been estimated that 50 HyCoSy procedures need to be performed before operators can be reasonably sure of their findings. A national teaching course is currently available.

Testicular structure and function

Ultrasound can be useful for locating ectopic testicles or in the diagnosis of testicular or epididymal tumours, but there is a poor correlation between testicular function and structural findings within the testicle. Hence it is not used routinely in the investigation of male subfertility. Small varicoceles, although detectable with ultrasound, do not lead to improved fertility when they are treated surgically, so a routine search for them is unjustified.

Ovulation induction

Ultrasound is ideal for monitoring the response of the ovary to stimulatory drugs for all the reasons previously mentioned. Frequent blood sampling for oestradiol levels used to be used but this is now rarely necessary.

For women who do not ovulate spontaneously, drugs such as clomifene stimulate FSH from the pituitary gland and therefore stimulate follicle growth in the ovary. Alternatively FSH, which is available commercially in a variety of preparations, usually in combination with LH, can be given directly by injection. In these circumstances ultrasound is used to check the numbers of follicles developing on each ovary. If more than two preovulatory-sized follicles (≥ 16 mm diameter) develop, there is the chance of a multiple gestation of triplets or more and conception needs to be avoided. Follicles are usually measured in two planes, their longest diameter and the diameter at right angles to this. It is possible to rotate the vaginal transducer through 90% and measure a third diameter but this adds little to precision. What really matters is how quickly the follicles are growing and how many of them there are.

Ultrasound is often used to decide on the timing of an injection of human chorionic gonadotrophin in order to trigger ovulation. Depending on protocol and circumstances this may be when the leading follicle is 20 mm diameter. If the scan is repeated 48 hours later to confirm ovulation, the follicle should have ruptured and a small amount of fluid may be visible behind the uterus in the pouch of Douglas.

In vitro fertilisation

The first step in in vitro fertilisation (IVF) is to inhibit pharmacologically the secretion of the gonadotrophins FSH and LH from the pituitary gland. This is termed downregulation. Ultrasound is used to check that adequate downregulation has been obtained by checking that the ovaries have become inactive with no follicles greater than 9 mm diameter and that the endometrium is thin (< 4 mm), i.e. that the serum oestadiol is low.

Follicle growth is then monitored in much the same way as in ovulation induction but there is no risk of supermultiple gestations with IVF because all the oocytes are extracted from their follicles and only one or two embryos subsequently transferred to the uterus. Hence higher doses of drugs can be used and many more follicles develop. Multiple ovarian follicles often push together to give a cartwheel appearance.

Vaginal ultrasound is the method of choice for harvesting the oocytes unless an ovary is situated in an unusual intra-abdominal position. A needle is passed through a guide on the transducer, through the vaginal fornix and into the ovary on each side. Follicular fluid is aspirated and examined microscopically to find each oocyte. This is a relatively safe procedure, although there are instances of pelvic infection or damage to the internal iliac vein. The vein is immediately adjacent to the ovary and can look very much like a follicle in cross-section, so if there is any doubt a follicle should be scanned from wall to wall before puncture.

If the oocytes fertilise successfully in vitro they are usually transferred to the uterus 2 or 3 days after their collection. Ultrasound can be useful in assisting embryo transfer.[5] The objective here is to transfer the embryos through the cervical canal into the upper uterine cavity as quickly as possible and with minimal trauma. Ultrasound can record the length and direction of the cervical canal and uterine cavity prior to attempts at transfer so as to make the procedure easier.

Ovarian hyperstimulation syndrome

Ovarian hyperstimulation syndrome (OHSS) may develop in the first few days and weeks after oocyte capture if the ovaries have been inadvertently overstimulated. It is more common in women who have PCO syndrome (PCOS) and when more than 15 or 20 oocytes have been harvested. It is rare to see the syndrome except in IVF cycles, although it can occur after ovulation induction or even after spontaneous ovulation. Women complain of abdominal pain and distension, nausea, diarrhoea and sometimes breathlessness. They retain fluid within the peritoneal and thoracic cavities and hence urine output falls, blood viscosity increases and there is a risk of venous thromboembolism. Ultrasound appearances help to differentiate the syndrome into mild, moderate and severe cases. Ovaries are less than 5 cm in diameter in mild cases, between 5 and 12 cm in moderate cases and greater than 12 cm in severe cases. There is also an increasing amount of intraperitoneal fluid in the more severe forms, most notably adjacent to the kidneys.

OHSS can be avoided by abandoning treatment prior to the human chorionic gonadotrophin ovulatory trigger in cases where a large number of follicles are seen to be developing. Alternatively, if oocyte capture has already taken place, all resulting embryos can be cryopreserved and not transferred to the uterus until the condition has subsided. This avoids pregnancy, which potentiates the condition.

Of course abdominal pain after embryo transfer has many other causes. Apart from OHSS the most serious of these is ectopic pregnancy. This can be a difficult diagnosis after IVF for a number of reasons. Human chorionic gonadotrophin is given as an ovulatory trigger so all women will have a positive pregnancy test for the first week or two after embryo transfer. The diagnosis of early pregnancy is often made before an intrauterine embryo is large enough to be seen. OHSS can occur at the same time as an ectopic. Even if an intrauterine embryo is seen, there may be a coincident tubal gestation (heterotopic pregnancy) as both the transferred embryos may have implanted. Suspicious cases may need to be followed by serial scans and serum beta – human chorionic gonadotrophin estimations. Miscarriages and molar pregnancies occur at least as commonly after IVF as after natural conception.

Doppler studies of follicles and endometrium

Advanced ultrasound techniques, although rarely used in clinical practice, have been used to enhance our knowledge of reproductive physiology. Doppler studies have shown increased blood flow around follicles with mature oocytes[6] and the pulsatility index of the endometrium correlates inversely with the probability of implantation.[7]

Uterine contractions

The uterine endometrium is in a constant state of movement throughout most of the menstrual cycle. However movements are slow and can only be demonstrated by speeding up video recordings of vaginal ultrasound images. Using this technique peristaltic-like waves can be seen to run along the length of the uterus in either direction and occasionally laterally towards the fallopian-tube orifices. A typical wave progresses along the uterus at a speed of about 3 cm/min. Contractions are more frequent at the time of ovulation in natural cycles or at the time of oocyte collection in IVF cycles. These contractions are thought to have a function in both sperm transport[8] and in implantation[9] and in the future their monitoring may have important implications for the management of subfertile couples. We know, for example, that the high incidence of ectopic pregnancy (4%) after IVF treatment is probably caused by uterine contractions relocating the embryos from the uterine cavity to the fallopian tubes.[10] A traumatic embryo transfer increases endometrial contractions and reduces the chances of pregnancy.[11]

Polycystic ovary syndrome

PCO are a common finding. The original ultrasonic definition calls for an enlarged ovary with more than 10 follicles up to 8 mm in diameter situated peripherally around an echo-dense, thickened central stroma.[12] Using this definition some 23% of ovaries were said to appear polycystic,[13] but the greater resolving power of modern vaginal transducers detects more follicles and therefore includes even more women in the diagnosis. A PCO, as an isolated ultrasound finding, has no relevance for fertility.[14] However, when combined with other symptoms of the PCOS, such as obesity, hirsutism or irregular periods, women with PCO are increasingly subfertile.

Women with PCOS may respond to ovulation induction by producing multiple preovulatory follicles and there is therefore a greater risk of supermultiple gestations. The diagnosis of PCOS is, therefore, an important one for ultrasonographers to note. It is also important to note, from a physiological point of view, that these ovaries are constantly changing. The follicles seen one day become atretic and are replaced by others by the time a scan is repeated a week later, even though the overall ovarian appearance is unaltered.

Pelvic pathology

It is not uncommon for pelvic pathology to be completely asymptomatic apart from its effect on fertility and hence to present for the first time during fertility investigations. Examples would be uterine malformations, endometriosis, uterine fibroids or hydrosalpinges. The latter three conditions may be hormone-dependent and increase in size in response to superovulation during IVF treatment. Occasionally they seem to appear for the first time during treatment, having been missed at a baseline scan when they were smaller.

REFERENCES

1. M. A. M. Hassan and S. R. Killick, Effect of male age on fertility: evidence for the decline in male fertility with increasing age. *Fertility and Sterility*, **79** (suppl. 3) (2003), 1520–7.

2. M. G. R. Hull, C. M. Glazener, N. J. Kelly, *et al.* Population study of causes, treatment, and outcome of infertility. *British Medical Journal*, **291** (1985), 1693–7.

3. *NICE Clinical Guideline. Fertility: Assessment and Treatment for People with Fertility Problems* (NICE, 2004).

4. S. R. Killick, Hysterosalpingo contrast sonography as a screening test for tubal patency in infertile women. *Journal of the Royal Society of Medicine*, **92** (1999), 628–31.

5. F. P. Biervliet, P. Lesny, S. D. Maguiness and S. R. Killick, Ultrasound-guided embryo transfer maximizes the IVF results on day 3 and day 4 embryo transfer but has no impact on day 5. *Human Reproduction*, **17** (2002), 1131.

6. G. Nargund, T. Bourne, P. Doyle *et al.*, Associations between ultrasound indices of follicular blood flow, oocyte recovery and preimplantation oocyte quality. *Human Reproduction*, **11** (1996), 109–13.

7. J. Zaidi, R. Pittrof, A. Shaker *et al.*, Assessment of uterine artery blood flow on the day of human chorionic gonadotropin administration by transvaginal color Doppler ultrasound in an in vitro fertilization program. *Fertility and Sterility*, **65** (1996), 377–81.

8. M. Fukuda and K. Fukuda, Uterine endometrial cavity movement and cervical mucus. *Human Reproduction*, **9** (1994), 1013–16.

9. M. M. Ijland, J. L. H. Evers, G. A. J. Dunselman *et al.*, Relation between endometrial wavelike activity and fecundability in spontaneous cycles. *Fertility and Sterility*, **67** (1997), 492–5.

10. F. P. Biervliet, P. Lesny, S. D. Maguiness and S. R. Killick, Mechanisms for bilateral ectopics after embryo transfer? *Fertility and Sterility*, **76** (2001), 212–13.

11. P. Lesny, S. R. Killick, J. Robinson, G. Raven and S. D. Maguiness, Junctional zone contractions and embryo transfer: is it safe to use a tenaculum? *Human Reproduction*, **14** (1999), 2367–70.

12. J. Adams, S. Franks, D. W. Polson *et al.*, Multifollicular ovaries: clinical and endocrine features and response to pulsatile gonadotropin releasing hormone. *Lancet*, **ii** (1985), 1375–8.

13. D. W. Polson, J. Wadsworth, J. Adams and S. Franks, Polycystic ovaries: a common finding in normal women. *Lancet*, **i** (1988), 870–2.

14. M. A. Hassan and S. R. Killick, Ultrasound diagnosis of polycystic ovaries in women who have no symptoms of polycystic ovary syndrome is not associated with subfecundity or subfertility. *Fertility and Sterility*, **80** (2003), 966–97.

8

Paediatric gynaecological ultrasound

David W. Pilling MB ChB DCH DMRD FRCR FRCPCH

Royal Liverpool Children's Hospital, Alder Hey, Liverpool

Ultrasound is clearly established as the imaging modality of choice for the evaluation of paediatric gynaecological conditions. In certain circumstances magnetic resonance imaging (MRI) will also have a role, as will specialised techniques such as genitography. Computed tomography (CT) has a very limited place and should be avoided, if possible, because of the significant dose of ionising radiation to the ovaries.

Ultrasound technique

Children of all ages have many special needs and all ultrasound examinations should be undertaken by those with experience of managing children who are also aware of the very different pathology likely to be encountered. Particularly for smaller children, a friendly environment is essential with appropriate toys and books to distract especially the preschool child.

As scans must be carried out transabdominally, a full bladder is necessary, which most girls over the age of 3 or 4 years can readily achieve. In younger children and babies it is pure chance as to whether the bladder is full or not. If it is not, then the infant should be given a drink and rescanned at half-hourly intervals until the bladder is full enough for an adequate examination. In neonates the bladder tends to fill and empty even more quickly so the time interval can be shorter.

Modern broadband curvilinear transducers are most appropriate, with a frequency range of 5–8 MHz in the neonate, 4–7 MHz in the older child and 3–5 MHz reserved for adolescents. In the neonate a linear 5–10 MHz probe (perhaps surprisingly) can occasionally be very useful, as the structures of interest are always within 1–2 cm of the probe and the linear configuration is not as big a handicap as may at first be thought.

In the USA transvaginal sonography in the appropriate clinical situations is undertaken in sexually active adolescents. This is not generally the practice in the UK.

Normal anatomy

The uterus and ovaries undergo significant changes between birth and puberty and these must be appreciated in order to avoid misinterpreting normal changes as pathological processes.[1] At birth both the uterus and ovaries are affected by maternal and placental gonadotrophins and as this stimulus disappears, so their appearances change over the first few months. Further significant changes take place at the time of puberty. A chart of normal measurements with age is essential.

Neonates and young infants

At birth the fundal region of the uterus is proportionately larger than at a slightly older age. The length of

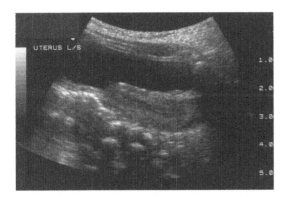

Figure 8.1 Neonatal uterus showing prominent endometrium with multiple layers due to maternal hormone stimulus.

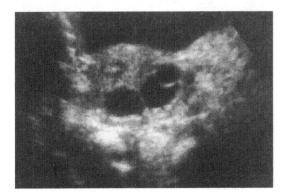

Figure 8.2 Normal ovary at 1 month with volume of 0.9 cm^3 and small microcysts.

the uterus is between 2.3 and 4.0 cm and the width between 0.8 and 2.2 cm. The endometrium may be visualised as an echogenic stripe and there may be a little fluid within the endometrial cavity (Fig. 8.1).

By birth the ovaries have usually descended to lie at the superior margin of the broad ligament, although rarely they may be as high as the lower pole of the kidneys. On ultrasound they appear homogeneous apart from the frequent presence of small microcysts (Fig. 8.2). Mean ovarian volume has been shown to be 1.06 cm^3 (range 0.7–3.6 cm^3) up to 3 months of age; 1.05 cm^3 (range 0.2–2.7 cm^3) in girls aged 4–12 months; and 0.67 cm^3 (range 0.1–1.7 cm^3) in girls between 13 and 24 months old.[1] The uterus in particular is very easy to demonstrate at this age – more

Table 8.1 Paediatric uterine and ovarian growth

Age	Uterine length (mm)[a]			Ovarian volume (cm^3)		
	Mean		SD	Mean		SD
2	33.1	±	4.4	0.75	±	0.41
4	32.9	±	3.3	0.82	±	0.36
6	33.2	±	4.1	1.19	±	0.36
8	35.8	±	7.3	1.05	±	0.50
10	40.3	±	6.4	2.22	±	0.69
12	54.3	±	8.4	3.80	±	1.40
13	53.8	±	11.4	4.18	±	2.30

[a] Total uterine length from fundus to cervix.
Data from Orsini *et al.*[40]

so than at any stage between 1 month and puberty. For this reason it is imperative to scan babies with ambiguous genitalia at this age rather than later in infancy. The ovaries are easily identified if follicles are present but more difficult if not.

Premenarchal girls

Beyond the neonatal period the uterus assumes a more tubular or teardrop shape with the cervix accounting for two-thirds of the total length (Fig. 8.3). The length of the uterus and the size of the ovaries change very little in the first 6 years of life but then gradually increase (Table 8.1). Throughout this time small microcysts within the ovaries may be seen on ultrasound scanning (Fig. 8.4) but it may be difficult to demonstrate normal ovaries at this age. By the age of 7 years the uterus has achieved a static phase which it maintains until the onset of puberty (Fig. 8.5).

Puberty

The uterus increases in size and changes shape at the time of puberty (Table 8.1), assuming a pear shape and starting to undergo cyclical endometrial changes identical to the adult. With gonadotrophin stimulus the ovaries enlarge and lie more deeply in the pelvis either laterally or posterolaterally to the uterus.

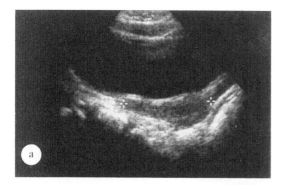

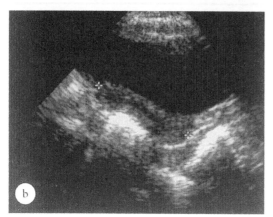

Figure 8.3 (a) At 6 months the cervix is more prominent than the fundus and body of the uterus. (b) By 1 year the uterus has assumed a more tubular appearance.

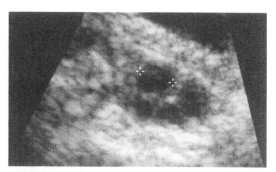

Figure 8.4 Normal ovary containing microcysts in a 3.5-year-old.

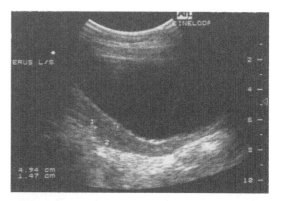

Figure 8.5 Normal uterus at 7 years of age with cervix more prominent than body.

Follicular development

Small (less than 0.9 cm) microcysts or follicles are frequently seen in the ovaries at any time between birth and puberty. They have been shown to occur in 84% of ovaries between birth and 2 years of age.[2] In the same study larger macrocysts (1–1.4 cm) were noted in 18% of normal ovaries. From 6 or 7 years onwards the number and size of cysts increase, although it is unusual for the cysts to be larger than 1.5 cm in diameter. In girls aged between 2 and 10 years, cysts up to 1.7 cm in diameter have been identified in 68%.[3]

At the time of puberty cyclical follicular development begins with a number of small primordial follicles being present early in the cycle. Between days 8 and 12 of the cycle a dominant follicle becomes apparent with ovulation occurring at mid-cycle when the follicle is between 1.7 and 2.7 cm in size. With follicular rupture the follicle decreases in size and a corpus luteum forms. This appears as a 1.6–2.4-cm cystic structure with internal echoes, which degenerates at the end of the cycle if fertilisation does not occur.

Neonatal pathology

Ovarian cysts

With the widespread use of both antenatal and post-natal ultrasound scanning, ovarian cysts of greater than 1.5 cm in diameter have been diagnosed

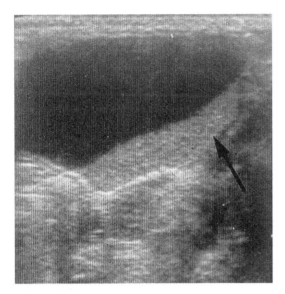

Figure 8.6 A 5-cm unilocular neonatal ovarian cyst with debris (arrow) in its base.

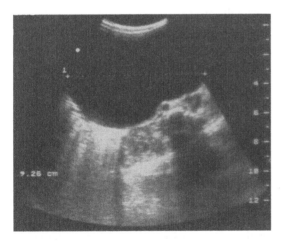

Figure 8.7 Large neonatal ovarian cyst about 9 cm in diameter. This resolved in infancy following partial aspiration.

with increasing frequency. Occasionally larger cysts present as abdominal masses or as bowel obstruction or respiratory embarrassment (Figs. 8.6 and 8.7). In these cases absolute differentiation from other cystic structures such as mesenteric, duplication or urachal cysts can be extremely difficult, although the pres-

ence of a daughter cyst is virtually pathognomonic.[4] All ovarian cysts can theoretically undergo torsion or cyst rupture, although this is unusual with the small ones.

Most neonatal ovarian cysts are of follicular origin. The stimulus to cyst formation is thought to be maternal gonadotrophins leading to aberrant follicular development. It is therefore reasonable to assume that after birth, when this stimulus is removed, at least some of these cysts will resolve. As a result of this a conservative approach to their management has been advocated. There is no agreement on the frequency of scanning but it seems reasonable to scan weekly in the first few weeks of life with less frequent scans as the baby gets older and the cyst reduces in size. Residual cysts can be seen up to 9 months of age and possibly longer. If a cyst increases in size or fails to involute, the diagnosis of follicular cyst should be questioned. Early studies suggested that only uncomplicated cysts which were totally anechoic and thin-walled should be managed in this way and that other complicated cysts should be removed. More recent studies have shown that most asymptomatic cysts can be managed conservatively with serial ultrasound monitoring.[5] Symptomatic cysts can be treated by percutaneous aspiration or surgery. Minilaparotomy has been suggested,[6] as has laparoscopy.[7] It has always been the surgical practice to conserve the ovaries in the rare situation of bilateral ovarian cysts but ovarian conservation is encouraged even with unilateral cysts wherever possible. The ultrasound appearances of complicated cysts include the presence of fluid/debris levels, retracting clot, septa or calcification in the cyst wall, but neither these features nor the size reliably predict the clinical outcome (Fig. 8.6).[8]

Vaginal bleeding

Neonatal vaginal bleeding is an uncommon event, usually caused by shedding of the endometrium which has become hypertrophied in utero secondary to maternal hormone stimulus and following removal of the stimulus behaves in the same way that the adult endometrium does. Ultrasound will show a prominent midline echo sometimes with a low echo element. Reassurance can be given in the presence of a normal-size uterus and lack of demonstrable ovarian pathology. Follow-up scans are only justified if the bleeding continues.

Hydrocolpos or hydrometrocolpos

Vaginal obstruction in the neonate may lead to fluid secretions distending the vagina (hydrocolpos) or the vagina and uterus (hydrometrocolpos).[9] This may be due to imperforate hymen, complete vaginal membrane, vaginal stenosis or atresia. More rarely it may be associated with a urogenital sinus or cloacal malformation. Urogenital sinus is a condition in which there is a single opening for the bladder and vagina whereas with a cloacal malformation there is a single perineal opening for the bladder, vagina and rectum. These types of abnormality are often also associated with other congenital anomalies such as bicornuate uterus, imperforate anus, oesophageal or duodenal atresia, congenital heart disease or renal abnormalities.

The fluid distension of the vagina and/or uterus leads to a predominantly cystic tubular midline mass lying between the bladder and rectum (Fig. 8.8). The fluid within this mass often contains low-level echoes due to the presence of debris. Occasionally the mass may be very large, containing up to 1 litre of fluid and, if very large, may displace the bladder, causing ureteric obstruction and even hydronephrosis.

Ambiguous genitalia

Rapid and accurate assessment of a newborn with ambiguous genitalia is required so that a decision can be made as to whether the child should be brought up as a boy or a girl.[10,11] The main role of ultrasound is to determine whether a uterus is present. As the uterus is most easily seen in the neonatal period the examination should be undertaken as soon as possible after birth. Whilst the changes on ultrasound will be clearly visible for several weeks after birth the examination should be undertaken with a degree of urgency because of the inevitable parental anxiety

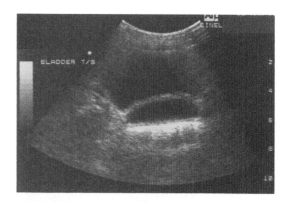

Figure 8.8 Transverse section of bladder with fluid-filled vagina behind. This is usually of no pathological significance.

this distressing situation causes. In later childhood transrectal ultrasound may play a role in the detailed assessment of the pelvis.[12] As well as ultrasound, genitography (the introduction of a contrast medium into the presumed vagina) is often also required to define the presence or absence of a vagina or urogenital sinus. Sex assignment is based on a combination of chromosomal analysis, gonadal biopsy and the knowledge of genital anatomy. Surgical management and its timing remain controversial.[13]

Ambiguous genitalia may be classified into four main groups: (1) female intersex (female pseudohermaphroditism); (2) true hermaphroditism; (3) mixed gonadal dysgenesis; and (4) male intersex (male pseudohermaphroditism).[14]

Female intersex is seen in females with normal chromosomes (46 XX). These babies have masculinised external genitalia with an enlarged clitoris, prominent fused labia and an elongated male-type urethra. The usual cause is excessive androgenic stimulus and this is often the result of congenital adrenal hyperplasia. These babies have normal female internal genital anatomy.

True hermaphrodites usually have an ovary on one side and a testis on the other side or the gonads may be fused as ovotestes. A uterus is often present but may be hypoplastic.

In mixed gonadal dysgenesis there is asymmetric gonadal differentiation, often with both a testis and a streak gonad. A uterus is usually present.

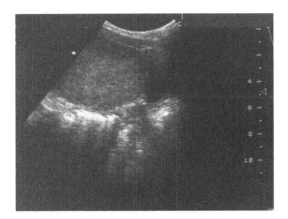

Figure 8.9 Solid pelvic tumour superior to the bladder. Histologically this was a rhabdomyosarcoma.

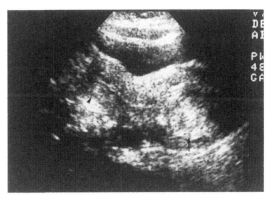

Figure 8.10 Vaginal rhabdomyosarcoma (arrow) abutting the uterus (arrowhead) in a 5-month-old girl with vaginal bleeding.

In male intersex (male pseudohermaphroditism) there are testes with feminisation or ambiguous external genitalia with an XY karyotype. Ultrasound is required to evaluate the presence or absence of gonads and a uterus. Congenital androgen insensitivity is probably the commonest cause of this rare situation.

Abnormalities in premenarchal girls

Vaginal bleeding/discharge

In the absence of evidence of pubertal development vaginal bleeding and/or discharge will often justify an ultrasound of the pelvis. It is however also important to exclude a foreign body as the cause of this symptom by examination which will probably need to be undertaken under anaesthetic. Ultrasound rarely demonstrates vaginal foreign bodies but has a role in excluding tumours such as rhabdomyosarcoma which, although rare, can present in this way (Fig. 8.9).

A rhabdomyosarcoma usually arises from the anterior vaginal wall adjacent to the cervix. It can occasionally infiltrate the uterus or arise primarily from within the uterus itself. These tumours appear on ultrasound as inhomogeneous solid masses lying behind the bladder in the region of the vagina and cervix (Fig. 8.10). They usually present in children

under the age of 5 with vaginal bleeding or polypoid prolapse of the tumour through the vagina. They need to be differentiated from vaginal adenocarcinoma, which is extremely rare.

Occasionally vaginal discharge is due to urine draining into the vagina from an ectopic ureter so that it may be helpful to assess the kidneys by ultrasound in this group of girls.

Precocious puberty

Precocious puberty is the appearance of gonadal maturation or secondary sexual characteristics before 8 years of age in girls and 9.5 years in boys. Isosexual precocious puberty refers to pubertal manifestations which are appropriate to the sex of the child. For example, premature breast development in a female is considered isosexual. If the pubertal manifestation is inappropriate for the child's sex (e.g. virilisation occurring in a girl) then this is considered a heterosexual disorder.

Central precocious puberty

In girls the majority of cases are idiopathic with no cause found. MRI can however be useful where there is a demonstrable cause such as hydrocephalus and hamartomas producing gonadotrophins. Hamartomas can produce precocious puberty at a very early age even in the neonatal period. Precocious puberty can also follow severe brain injury or infection as well as being associated with neurofibromatosis, tuberous sclerosis and primary hypothyroidism.

The role of ultrasound including uterine artery Doppler[15] in the investigation of precocious puberty is to determine the size and degree of development of the uterus and ovaries[16, 17] as well as assessing the presence of ovarian cysts or masses. It may also be appropriate to evaluate the adrenal glands by ultrasound, CT or MRI and, in true precocious puberty, MRI of the brain is necessary.[18–20]

True precocious puberty is seen in association with increased oestrogen and gonadotrophin levels. There is enlargement of the uterus and ovaries with ovulation before the age of 8 years and the development of secondary sexual characteristics. Some 60–80% are due to idiopathic activation of the hypothalamic–pituitary–gonadal axis but in the others there may be a demonstrable abnormality of the central nervous system and hence the need for MRI scanning.

Pseudosexual precocity

This is more unusual and is characterised by finding raised sex hormones with normal gonadotrophin levels. The most frequent cause is a hormone-secreting ovarian tumour, although rarely an adrenal tumour may secrete these hormones and cause similar findings.

McCune–Albright syndrome can cause pubertal development independent of gonadotrophins but the mechanism is not well understood.

Premature thelarche and premature adrenarche

Premature thelarche is used to describe isolated breast development and, in its early stages, is difficult to differentiate from precocious puberty. Hormone profile is usually normal for early puberty and treatment is not usually necessary.

Premature adrenarche is the growth of pubic and axillary hair before the age of 8. It is due to elevation in adrenal androgens which are in the pubertal range but other investigations are normal. If late onset of

congenital adrenal hyperplasia is excluded no treatment is necessary.

Ultrasound of the pelvis and adrenal is sometimes requested in these situations and can be reassuring if normal, prepubertal appearances are seen.

A recent study looking at the usefulness of assessing ovarian volume and the presence of cysts in female isosexual precocious puberty has provided some helpful guidelines.[21] Bilateral ovarian enlargement (mean ovarian volume 4.6 cm^3) appears to be a reliable indicator of true precocious puberty whereas unilateral ovarian enlargement (mean volume 4.1 cm^3) in combination with macrocysts (greater than 9 mm in size) is suggestive of incomplete precocious puberty. In the same study looking at girls under the age of 8 years, mean ovarian volume in the control group and in a small group with premature adrenarche was less than 1 cm^3. Although microcysts (less than 9 mm in diameter) can be seen in normal ovaries at all ages it has been suggested that these microcysts are seen more frequently and are more numerous in girls with isolated premature thelarche.[22]

Hirsutism

This is an embarrassing condition which is age- and race-dependent. Hair growth is androgen-dependent and is therefore associated with excess androgens or excessive response to normal levels. In the paediatric age group it is associated with polycystic ovary syndrome, late-onset adrenal hyperplasia, obesity, ovarian or adrenal tumours, Cushing's syndrome or drugs. A proportion are idiopathic.

Gynaecological pelvic masses in premenarchal girls

These account for 3–4% of all abdominopelvic masses in children. Many are simple benign ovarian cysts which fulfil the ultrasound criteria for a cyst, usually being unilocular, thin-walled and totally anechoic. Occasionally, haemorrhage within a simple cyst may alter the appearances so that they are difficult to differentiate from solid ovarian masses. Serous cystadenomas or cystadenocarcinomas may

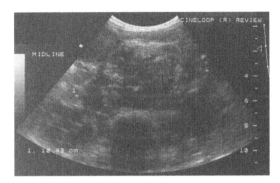

Figure 8.11 Transverse section of the lower abdomen showing a mixed echo mass which histologically proved to be a neuroblastoma.

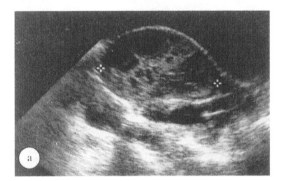

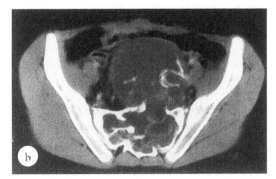

Figure 8.12 (a) Multi-loculated semicystic semisolid lesion in a 12-year-old girl with back pain. (b) Computed tomographic examination of the pelvis shows that this arises from the sacrum and is an aneurysmal bone cyst.

rarely occur in the ovaries of adolescents but are very rare before puberty. In the investigation of solid pelvic masses the primary role of ultrasound is to

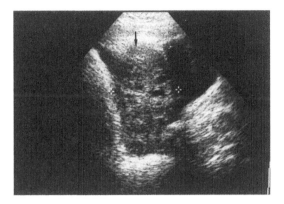

Figure 8.13 Predominantly solid ovarian dysgerminoma lying in the midline of the pelvis in a 10-year-old girl.

identify the organ of origin. Many of the solid masses that can occur in the pelvis have similar appearances and can be very difficult to differentiate. Although many of the masses will arise from the ovaries, it is important to remember that others such as neuroblastoma, sacrococcygeal teratoma, lymphadenopathy, bowel-related lesions, abscesses (particularly related to the appendix) and pelvic inflammatory disease may occur (Fig. 8.11). Some of these may mimic cystic ovarian masses (Fig. 8.12). Other imaging modalities such as MRI and CT may aid differentiation. Rhabdomyosarcomas may also present as a pelvic mass throughout childhood. These arise from the vagina in this age group. They may also present as a mass at the introitus.

Ovarian tumours

About a third of these are malignant. The most common ovarian tumour is a teratoma (or dermoid cyst) which is usually, but not always, benign, with the most common malignant tumour being a dysgerminoma (Figs. 8.13 and 8.14). The most common tumour to be seen in association with precocious puberty is a granulosa thecal cell tumour (Fig. 8.15). Other rare causes of ovarian masses are fibromas which can be associated with pleural effusions (Meigs syndrome) and leukaemic infiltration.[23,24]

Teratomas can occur in both pre- and postpubertal girls but are more common after puberty. They may

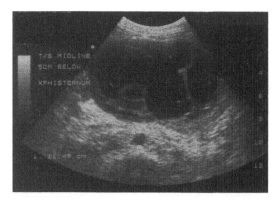

Figure 8.14 Mixed cystic and solid tumour. Histologically this proved to be a malignant teratoma.

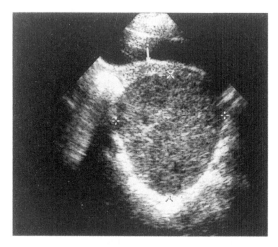

Figure 8.15 A 6.5-cm solid fairly homogeneous mass lying behind the uterus (arrow) in a 6-year-old and shown at surgery to be an ovarian juvenile granulosa cell tumour.

present due to the presence of a mass or as a result of torsion. Their appearances are varied. They often have hyper- and hypoechoic elements and may contain sebum, fat, hair and teeth. If the fat content is significant they may be overlooked on ultrasound as the echogenicity of the fat may be misinterpreted as adjacent bowel. The most characteristic findings are the presence of mural nodules and acoustic shadowing from teeth or calcification within a complex, solid and cystic mass (Fig. 8.16).[25] Clinically, recurrence of these tumours, if mature histologically, is unlikely

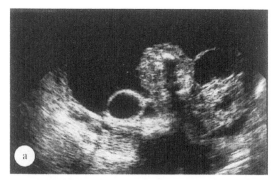

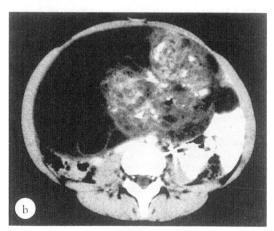

Figure 8.16 (a) An 11-year-old girl with a huge abdominopelvic teratoma shown on ultrasound to be a combination of cystic and solid areas with focal areas of calcification. (b) Computed tomography confirms the semisolid semicystic nature of the tumour as well as showing the extensive focal calcification within.

and regimens for follow-up used in adults can safely be used in children.[26] From the clinical viewpoint it is crucial that measurements in two planes are given to allow the clinician to appreciate the overall size of the lesion. It is impossible to give a confident histological diagnosis but a gynaecologist is likely to observe a small otherwise innocent-looking lesion but remove a larger one.

Pelvic pain

This is a common problem in girls; a gynaecological cause is unusual prepuberty. Adnexal torsion,

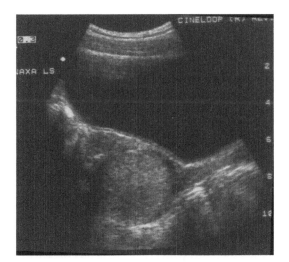

Figure 8.17 Longitudinal section showing a haemorrhagic ovarian cyst which is of uniform echogenicity.

which is more common after puberty, can also occur before.

Adnexal torsion presents with acute or intermittent abdominal or pelvic pain, which may be confused with conditions such as appendicitis and other common causes of abdominal pain in children, such as mesenteric adenitis. Normal adnexal structures, which in young girls are unusually mobile, may undergo torsion or there may be torsion of an ovarian mass. The degree of torsion is variable, ranging from lymphatic obstruction through venous obstruction to arterial occlusion. This leads to a markedly enlarged and oedematous ovary which, if completely infarcted, will show no blood flow on colour Doppler. The appearances may be misinterpreted as those of an ovarian tumour (Fig. 8.17). Occasionally a characteristic appearance of distended follicles on the surface of an abnormally enlarged ovary may give the clue to the diagnosis. A study of 20 girls, 11 of whom were prepubertal, showed a variety of appearances.[27] Neonates and young children with torsion were more likely to have extrapelvic cystic or complex cystic masses, whereas pubertal girls had predominantly solid masses in an adnexal location. Colour Doppler signals were fre-

quently detected in the torted ovaries, with absent flow in about a third of cases.

Ultrasound imaging of adolescent gynaecological problems

Problems with menstruation

Problems with menstruation are very common in adolescence.

Primary amenorrhoea is defined as the failure to menstruate by the age of 16. Gonadotrophin hormones (luteinising and follicle-stimulating hormone) stimulate the graafian follicle within the ovary, leading to ovulation. Following ovulation the corpus luteum produces oestrogen and progesterone, which prepares the endometrium for implantation. If fertilisation does not occur the blood levels of oestrogen and progesterone fall and the endometrium breaks down and menstruation ensues. Any interruption in this pathway may cause problems with menstruation. Abnormalities in the region of the pituitary or hypothalamus may be detected by MRI and rarely the cause may relate to androgen-producing tumours of the adrenal gland, which may be visualised with ultrasound or CT. Primary amenorrhoea may be further subdivided into those with otherwise normal secondary sex development and those who remain prepubertal. The role of ultrasound is to evaluate the presence of the uterus, ovaries and vagina and to assess whether they appear prepubertal or pubertal in size and shape in addition to detecting genital tract obstruction.[18]

Genital tract obstruction

Uterovaginal obstruction usually becomes apparent at puberty when the onset of menstruation leads to an accumulation of menstrual blood and secondary distension of the vagina (haematocolpos) (Fig. 8.18). In addition the uterus may also be distended (haematometrocolpos) (Fig. 8.19) or, rarely, the uterus alone is distended (haematometra). This distension may lead to cyclical lower abdominal pain without menstruation occurring.

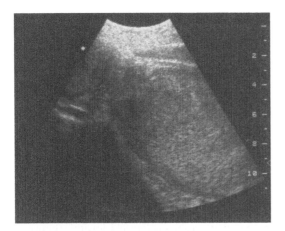

Figure 8.18 Soft-tissue mass of uniform density typical of haematometrocolpos. The uterus distended with blood products is seen at the left of the image.

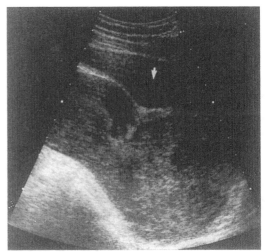

Figure 8.20 A pelvic abscess from a perforated appendix lying behind the bladder (arrow) in an 11-year-old girl mimicking haematometrocolpos.

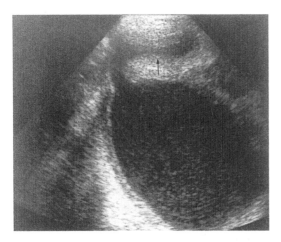

Figure 8.19 Echogenic fluid distension of the vagina with less distension of the uterus (arrow) in a 13-year-old girl with haematometrocolpos.

Three main types of uterovaginal abnormalities have been described[28] and the corresponding ultrasound findings documented.[29]

1. disorders of vertical fusion such as imperforate hymen, transverse vaginal septum and agenesis of the cervix
2. agenesis of the uterus and vagina (Mayer–Rokintansky–Kuster–Hauser syndrome). An active Müllerian duct remnant with functioning endometrial tissue may lead to unilateral haematometra
3. disorders of lateral fusion, usually leading to unilateral obstruction

The ultrasound appearances of haematocolpos and haematometrocolpos are of a tubular semifluid collection lying in the midline of the pelvis behind the bladder. The degree of internal echogenicity is variable and on occasions the mass may appear solid.

Confusion can arise with other pelvic fluid collections such as abscesses (Fig. 8.20). Infrequently a single horn of a bicornuate uterus or one part of a duplicated vagina may become obstructed and in this situation a similar pelvic mass is present but with normal menstruation (Fig. 8.21).

It must be remembered that in some cases of unilateral obstruction a confusing clinical picture presents with the ultrasound appearances of obstruction but with apparently normal periods. It is important to consider this diagnosis with any pelvic mass in this age group.[30–32]

Primary amenorrhoea with absence of sexual characteristic development

Any girl without secondary sex characteristics at the age of 14 warrants investigation. The commoner causes are shown in Table 8.2.

Table 8.2 Common causes of primary amenorrhoea

Constitutional delay
Chronic illness
Absence of ovarian function
    Gonadal dysgenesis
    Ovarian failure
Hypothalamic–pituitary
    dysfunction

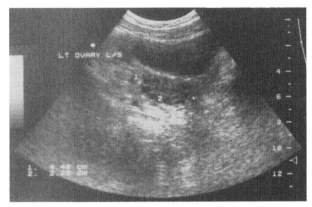

Figure 8.22 Longitudinal section of the ovary with multiple small peripheral cysts. These features, together with clinical findings are consistent with polycystic ovary syndrome.

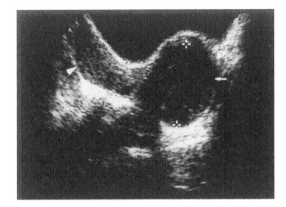

Figure 8.21 Unilateral haematocolpos (arrow) in a duplicated genital tract in a teenage girl with lower abdominal pain but normal menstruation. The normal right moiety of the genital tract can also be seen (arrowhead).

In girls with constitutional delay there is delay in maturation of the hypothalamic–pituitary–ovarian axis. Growth, bone age and sexual characteristics are all delayed. There is sometimes a history of such delay in other family members. Any child who is affected by a chronic illness may suffer a delay in puberty which often responds when the illness is treated.

Gonadal dysgenesis

The most common form of gonadal dysgenesis is Turner's syndrome, an abnormality of sex chromosomes (XO). In Turner's syndrome the uterus is normal although it may remain prepubertal in size and shape. About two-thirds of patients will have no visible ovarian tissue or simply 'streak' ovaries. On ultrasound, streak ovaries are visualised as very small

confluent streaks of tissue in the expected region of the ovaries. One-third of patients will have 'non-streak' ovaries which have variable appearances on ultrasound. These range from small ovaries, sometimes containing minute cysts, to normal-looking ovaries.[33] The importance of this differentiation is that non-streak ovaries may retain a degree of function and in some cases spontaneous breast development and uterine enlargement may occur. Artificial induction of puberty and treatment with growth hormone[34] in these young women cause uterine growth which can be monitored by ultrasound.[35]

Other causes of ovarian failure

These are all rare and include chromosome abnormalities other than Turner's syndrome, iatrogenic causes, including surgery and radiotherapy of the pelvis, and, more rarely still, infection. Ultrasound appearances are those of a prepubertal uterus and ovaries which are small or impossible to identify.

Congenital androgen insensitivity syndrome (CAIS)

This syndrome, which is also known as testicular feminisation syndrome, is caused by internal organ insensitivity to androgens.

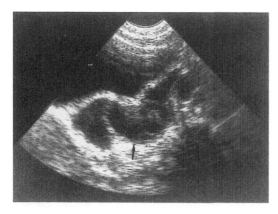

Figure 8.23 Dilated fluid-filled fallopian tube (arrow) in a teenage girl with pelvic inflammatory disease.

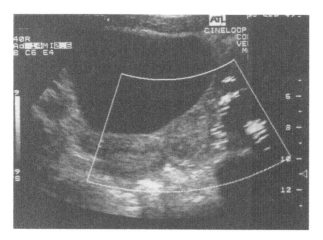

Figure 8.24 Transverse section of pelvis showing an inflammatory mass.

These patients have no uterus, a rudimentary vagina and testes lying somewhere between the retroperitoneum and the labia. They have a male karyotype and female phenotype.

Polycystic ovaries in childhood

Polycystic ovaries are a well-recognised cause of delayed puberty or menarche in teenage girls and this condition is considered later.

Secondary amenorrhoea

In teenage girls the most common cause of secondary amenorrhoea is pregnancy. Other causes include functional cysts, polycystic ovary syndrome or ovarian failure. Much rarer causes would be ovarian tumours or central nervous system lesions.

Polycystic ovary syndrome

This is a common cause of menstrual disturbance in adolescence. Polycystic ovary syndrome is characterised by luteinising-hormone oversecretion and hyperandrogenism. Disordered folliculogenesis results and this is seen in as many as 23% of the population.[35] The syndrome should only be diagnosed where menstrual disturbance, obesity, acne and hirsutism are found together with the appropriate hormone profile.[36, 37]

Menstrual disturbances include secondary amenorrhoea or menorrhagia (heavy periods). On ultrasound scanning these ovaries must be differentiated from the normally appearing multicystic ovaries that are seen before or during puberty. Multicystic ovaries are normal-sized ovaries containing more than six cysts measuring greater than 4 mm in diameter, but with a normal stromal pattern. Polycystic ovaries may be of normal or increased size and tend to have an excessive number of small, peripherally based cysts and an increased stromal pattern (Fig. 8.22). However, not all girls with polycystic ovaries will have polycystic ovary syndrome. Even in the absence of manifestations of the polycystic ovary syndrome there does appear to be an association between polycystic ovaries, obesity and a later reduction in fertility.[38]

Congenital abnormalities of the uterus

It may only be possible to detect these with ultrasound at or after puberty when the uterus has enlarged. Even then some of the minor abnormalities such as uterine and vaginal septa may be impossible to visualise.

The most common congenital abnormality is a bicornuate uterus where there is fusion which is confined to the caudal end of the Müllerian duct system. This leads to two uterine bodies joined at variable levels above the cervix. On ultrasound examination the uterus may be slightly wider than usual with two endometrial echoes from each cornual region which converge in the lower uterine body.[39]

Much less common is the finding of uterus didelphys where there is failure of fusion of the dual Müllerian duct system leading to two uteri, two cervices and two vaginas. Unilateral failure of Müllerian duct development is slightly more common, giving a uterus unicornis unicollis which, on ultrasound, appears as a smaller than normal uterine body with a single cervix and vagina.

Pelvic masses in adolescent girls

Many of these have been described in the section on premenarchal girls, above. With the onset of puberty the incidence of functional ovarian cysts, which may vary in size from 2 to 10 cm, increases greatly. These functional cysts may present as palpable masses or give pain due to torsion or rupture. They may be follicular, corpus luteal or theca lutein cysts. The latter cysts may be multiloculated and therefore confused with cystadenoma or even cystadenocarcinoma.

Pelvic pain

Gynaecological causes of pelvic pain include mid-cycle mittelschmerz pain, torsion or rupture of ovarian cysts, torsion of normal ovaries or ovarian masses, endometriosis, ectopic pregnancy and pelvic inflammatory disease (Figs. 8.23 and 8.24). The risk of pelvic inflammatory disease is increased in the young sexually active adolescent. The ultrasound findings of these conditions have either been described elsewhere in this chapter or are identical to those that have been well-described in the adult population. Non-gynaecological causes, such as appendicitis, need to be borne in mind and looked for when carrying out ultrasound examinations for acute lower abdominal pain.

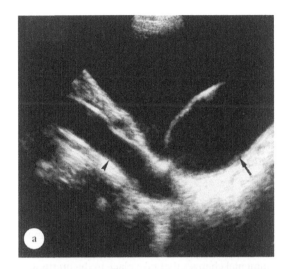

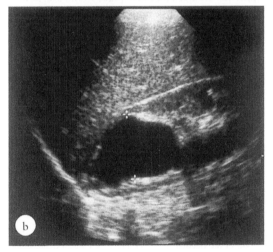

Figure 8.25 (a)Ureterocele within the bladder and associated hydroureter (arrowhead) in a newborn girl. (b) Further examination reveals an obstructed upper-pole moiety of a duplex kidney.

Associated renal tract abnormalities

It should be remembered that a number of congenital abnormalities of the genital tract are also associated with abnormalities of the renal tract and these should be looked for at the time of the ultrasound scan. These include renal agenesis, renal ectopia and horseshoe kidneys. When scanning the pelvis, abnormalities of the renal tract may cause confusion. Dilated tubular structures behind the bladder may be due to dilated ureters and cyst-like structures within the bladder may be due to ureteroceles. Both of these findings should lead to an examination of the kidneys to look for hydronephrosis and the presence of duplex collecting systems (Fig. 8.25). A bladder diverticulum may be misinterpreted as an adnexal cyst and a close look for a communication with the bladder should be made.

Conclusion

Ultrasound examination of the paediatric female pelvis requires a thorough knowledge of the developmental changes that take place in the uterus and ovaries between birth and puberty. It also requires knowledge of the various congenital abnormalities that may occur and their associations with abnormalities elsewhere within the abdomen. The main role of ultrasound in the evaluation of a pelvic mass is to define whether the mass is cystic or solid and its organ of origin. Many of the solid pelvic masses have similar ultrasound appearances and a specific pathological diagnosis cannot be made until the time of surgery or biopsy.

REFERENCES

1. L. Garel, J. Dubois, A. Grignon, D. Filiatrault and G. Van Vliet, US of the paediatric female pelvis: a clinical perspective. *Radiographics,* **21** (2001) 193–407.

2. H. L. Cohen, M. A. Shapiro, F. S. Mandel and M. L. Shapiro, Normal ovaries in neonates and infants: a sonographic study of 77 patients 1 day to 24 months old. *American Journal of Roentgenology,* **160** (1993), 583–6.

3. H. L. Cohen, P. Eisenberg, F. Mandel and J. O. Haller, Ovarian cysts are common in premenarchal girls: a sonographic study of 101 children 2–12 years old. *American Journal of Roentgenology,* **159** (1992), 89–91.

4. H. J. Lee, S. K. Woo, J. S. Kim and S. J. Suh, "Daughter cyst" sign: a sonographic finding of ovarian cysts in neonates, infants and young children. *American Journal of Roentgenology,* **174** (2000), 1013–15.

5. C. Muller-Leisse, U. Bick, K. Paulussen *et al.,* Ovarian cysts in the fetus and neonate – changes in sonographic pattern in the follow-up and their management. *Pediatric Radiology,* **22** (1992), 395–400.

6. F. Ferro, D. Iacobelli, A. Zaccara *et al.,* Exteriorisation – aspiration mini laparotomy for treatment of neonatal ovarian cyst. *Journal of Pediatric and Adolescent Gynecology,* **15** (2002), 205–7.

7. D. Tseng, T. J. Curran and M. L. Silen, Minimally invasive management of the pre natally torted ovarian cyst. *Journal of Pediatric Surgery,* **37** (2002), 1467–9.

8. C. Mittermayer, W. Blaicher, D. Grassauer *et al.,* Fetal ovarian cysts: development and neonatal outcome. *Ultraschall Medicine,* **24** (2003), 21–6.

9. A. Nussbaum, A. R. Blask, R. C. Sanders and J. P. Gearhart, Obstructed uterovaginal anomalies: demonstration with sonography. Part I. Neonates and infants. *Radiology,* **179** (1991), 79–83.

10. Y. Low and J. M. Hutson, Rules for clinical diagnosis in babies with ambiguous genitalia. *Journal of Paediatric Child Health,* **39** (2003), 406–13.

11. C. Sultan, F. Paris, C. Jeandel, S. Lumbroso and R. B. Galifer, Ambiguous genitalia in the new born. *Seminars in Reproductive Medicine,* **20** (2002), 181–8.

12. J. A. Blanco, C. Perez, M. Jimenez *et al.,* Usefulness of transrectal ultrasonography in the diagnosis of anomalies of intersexual conditions. *Cir Pediatr* **16** (2003), 86–9.

13. L. Rangecroft, Surgical management of ambiguous genitalia. *Archives of Disease in Childhood,* **88** (2003), 799–801.

14. C. Battaglia, G. Regnani, F. Mancini *et al.,* Pelvic sonography and uterine color Doppler analysis in the diagnosis of female precocious puberty. *Ultrasound in Obstetrics and Gynaecology,* **19** (2002), 386–91.

15. T. D. Allen, Disorders of sexual differentiation. In *Clinical Pediatric Urology,* ed. P. P., Kelalis, L. R. King and A. B. Belman (Philadelphia: Saunders, 1985), pp. 904–21.

16. C. Battaglia, F. Mancini, G. Regnani *et al.,* Pelvic ultrasound and color Doppler findings in different isosexual precocities. *Ultrasound in Obstetrics and Gynaecology,* **22** (2003), 277–83.

17. L. D. Herter, E. Golendziner, J. A. Flores *et al.,* Ovarian and uterine findings in pelvic sonography: comparison between prepubertal girls, girls with isolated thelarche, and girls with central precocious puberty. *Journal of Ultrasound Medicine,* **21** (2002), 1237–46.

18. W. J. Zwiebel and K. A. Murray, Imaging assessment of pubertal disorders. *Seminars in Ultrasound, CT and MRI,* **16** (1995), 296–303.

19. S. M. Ng, Y. Kumar, D. Cody, C. S. Smith and M. Didi, Cranial MRI scans are indicated in all girls with central precocious puberty. *Archives of Disease in Childhood*, **88** (2003), 414–18.

20. A. Cassio, E. Cacciari, S. Zucchini *et al.*, Central precocious puberty: clinical and imaging aspects. *Journal of Pediatric Endocrinological Metabolism*, **13** (suppl. 1), (2000) 703–6.

21. L. R. King, M. J. Siegel and A. L. Solomon, Usefulness of ovarian volume and cysts in female isosexual precocious puberty. *Journal of Ultrasound Medicine*, **12** (1993), 577–81.

22. S. M. Freedman, P. M. Kreitzer, S. S. Elkowitz *et al.*, Ovarian microcysts in girls with isolated premature thelarche. *Journal of Pediatrics*, **122** (1993), 246–9.

23. J. L. Breen and W. S. Maxson, Ovarian tumours in children and adolescents. *Clinics in Obstetrics and Gynecology*, **20** (1977), 607–23.

24. A. Wu and M. Siegel, Sonography of pelvic masses in children: diagnostic predictability. *American Journal of Roentgenology*, **148** (1987), 1199.

25. C. L. Sisler and M. J. Siegel, Ovarian teratomas: a comparison of the sonographic Appearance in prepubertal and postpubertal girls. *American Journal of Roentgenology*, **154** (1990), 139–41.

26. C. L. Templeman, S. P. Hertweck, J. P. Scheetz, S. E. Pearlman and M. E. Fallat, The management of mature cystic teratomas in children and adolescents: a retrospective analysis. *Human Reproduction*, 15 (2000), 266–72.

27. J. E. Stark and M. J. Siegel, Ovarian torsion in prepubertal and pubertal girls: sonographic findings. *American Journal of Roentgenology*, **163** (1994), 1479–82.

28. J. A. Rock, Anomalous development of the vagina. *Seminars in Reproductive Endocrinology*, **4** (1986), 13–31.

29. A. R. Nussbaum Blask, R. C. Sanders and J. A. Rock, Obstructed uterovaginal anomalies: demonstration with sonography. part II. Teenagers. *Radiology*, **91**, 84–8.

30. L. Ballesio, C. Andreoli, M. L. De Cicco, Angeli and L. Mangananro, Haematocolpos in double vagina associated with uterus didelphus: US and MR findings. *European Journal of Radiology*, **45** (2003), 150–3.

31. S. Leurie, M. Feinstein and Y. Mamet, Unusual presentation of acute abdomen in a syndrome of double uterus, unilaterally imperforated double vagina and ipsilateral renal agenesis. *Acta Obstetrica Gynaecologica Scandinavica*, **79** (2000), 152–3.

32. C. Peironi, D. L. Rosenfeld and M. L. Mokrzycki, Uterus didelphys with obstructed hemivagina and ipspateral renal agenesis. A case report. *Journal of Reproductive Medicine*, **46** (2001), 133–6.

33. A. A. Massarono, J. A. Adams, M. A. Preece and C. G. D. Brook, Ovarian ultrasound appearances in Turner syndrome. *Journal of Pediatrics*, **114** (1989), 568–73.

34. P. Sampaolo, V. Calcaterra, C. Klersy *et al.*, Pelvic ultrasound evaluation in patients with Turner's syndrome during treatment with growth hormone. *Ultrasound in Obstetrics and Gynaecology*, **22** (2003), 172–7.

35. C. M. McDonnell, L. Coleman and M. R. Zacharin, A three year prospective study to assess uterine growth in girls with Turner's syndrome by pelvic ultrasound. *Clinics in Endocrinology (Oxford)*, **58** (2003), 446–50.

36. R. J. Norman, R. W. and M. T. Stankiewicz, Polycystic ovary syndrome. *Med J Aust*, **180** (2004) 132–7.

37. P. Sampaolo, C. Livieri, L. Montanari, *et al.*, Precocious signs of polycystic ovaries in obese girls. *Ultrasound in Obstetrics and Gynaecology*, **4** (1994), 3130–5.

38. C. G. D. Brook, H. S. Jacobs and R. Stanhope, Polycystic ovaries in childhood. *British Medical Journal*, **296** (1988), 878.

39. A. L. Deutch and B. B. Gosink, Non neoplastic gynecologic disorders. *Seminars in Roentgenology*, **17** (1982), 269–83.

40. L. F. Orisini, S. Salardi, G. Pilu, L. Bovicelli and E. Calliari, Pelvic organs in premenarchal girls real time ultrasonography. *Radiology*, **153** (1984), 113–16.

9

Clinical management of patients: the gynaecologist's perspective

Lynne Rogerson[1], Sean Duffy[1] and Chris Kremer[2]

[1] St James's University Hospital, Leeds
[2] Pinderfields General Hospital, Wakefield

Introduction

Probably the most significant contribution in the history of ultrasound within the field of obstetrics and gynaecology came from Professor Ian Donald at Glasgow in the early 1960s.[1] The types of pathology first identified in the uterus by pelvic ultrasonic scanning included hydatidiform moles[2] and retained products of conception.[3] Kratochwil[4] first described transvaginal ultrasonography in 1969, but it was only after its evaluation of infertility in the 1980s that its full potential was realised.[5] It is now also used in the investigation and management of infertility and assisted reproduction, early pregnancy,[6] tubal pregnancy[7] and first-trimester pregnancy-related conditions.

Clinical use of ultrasound in gynaecology

Why do gynaecologists request ultrasound scans? As in all clinical areas, examination skills are being lost or open to marked interobserver variation, resulting in greater reliance on investigations as a substitute. This opens up the abuse of such investigations with requests made with little thought as to how the investigation will help in diagnosis or management. Ultrasound should in no way replace physical examination; it should assist in building the clinical picture to contribute to appropriate patient management.

There are occasions, nevertheless, where the bimanual examination is just not enough. Obesity makes it more difficult to feel pelvic organs, and in such circumstances a transvaginal scan makes the pelvic organs more accessible. The patient may be virgo intacta and so pelvic examination is obviously inappropriate, or in a postmenopausal woman with atrophic tissues, examination may be very difficult or sometimes impossible due to discomfort. Ultrasound can also be used to reduce the use of more invasive investigations such as hysteroscopy or laparoscopy and may also reduce the chance of investigative major abdominal surgery.

From a clinical viewpoint the use of ultrasound can be roughly divided into pregnancy-related and non-pregnancy-related. In gynaecology, pregnancy-related topics usually refer to miscarriage (more properly referred to as early pregnancy loss) and ectopic pregnancy. Non-pregnancy-related clinical conditions range from lost intrauterine contraceptive devices through to postmenopausal bleeding. This chapter will concentrate on non-pregnancy-related clinical situations and helps to put into a clinical context the use of ultrasound in daily practice.

Non-pregnancy-related gynaecological conditions

It is perhaps easier to consider the need and practical use of ultrasound in gynaecology when one

Table 9.1 Causes of abnormal uterine bleeding

Organic	Iatrogenic
Uterine	Intrauterine contraceptive
Fibroids	device
Endometriosis	Anticoagulants
Adenomyosis	Progesterones
Endometrial/cervical polyps	Obesity
Pelvic inflammatory disease	
Endometrial hyperplasia/	
malignancy	
Coagulopathies	
Congenital deficiencies	
Thrombocytopenia	
Leukaemia	
Systemic disorders	
Hypothyroidism	
Systemic lupus	
erythematosis	
Chronic liver failure	

Table 9.2 Causes of postmenopausal bleeding

Gynaecological (96%)	Non-gynaecological (4%)
Malignant (12%)	Per rectum or per urethram
Primary tumours	bleeding, from
Secondary tumours	gastrointestinal or
Benign (88%)	genitourinary tract
Atrophic genital changes	pathology, may be mistaken
Exogenous/endogenous	for per vaginam bleeding in
Oestrogen	a minority of cases
Benign tumours	
Infection	
Injuries	

considers the symptom groups that are encountered. In broad terms, gynaecological patients requiring ultrasound fall into four main categories: (1) those with symptoms relating to 'period problems' (abnormal uterine bleeding: AUB); (2) symptoms relating to infertility; (3) symptoms or signs relating to a pelvic mass; and (4) pelvic pain. By far the commonest condition seen by gynaecologists is menstrual disorders.

Abnormal uterine bleeding

AUB can be divided into three main groups: (1) regular or irregular heavy bleeding (menorrhagia/metrorrhagia); (2) intermenstrual bleeding (IMB); and (3) postmenopausal bleeding (PMB), which includes abnormal bleeding on hormone replacement therapy (HRT).

There are many causes of AUB, ranging from organic to iatrogenic (Table 9.1). Once these are excluded in the premenopausal woman, a diagnosis of dysfunctional uterine bleeding (DUB) remains. In the postmenopausal group, 96% will have a gynaecological cause for the PMB and the remainder are non-gynaecological[8] (Table 9.2).

Premenopausal patients

Changes in women's lifestyles through the generations have meant that they are having fewer children, are breast-feeding for shorter intervals and frequently have busier lives trying to balance a family life and a career. Women therefore have more periods than previous generations, are less tolerant of them and seek advice more often. AUB, occurring before the menopause, accounts for nearly a third of referrals to a gynaecologist. The pattern of bleeding may be excessive heaviness, losing clots, with or without flooding each month, or a totally chaotic cycle with no pattern at all.

In premenopausal women the need to investigate the uterus is because of the likelihood of finding significant intrauterine pathology which may be the cause of the bleeding. Once found, fibroids and polyps can be treated in the hope of resolving the symptoms. Women who do not have an organic cause for the bleeding, that is, no pathological basis, are classified as having DUB.

The traditional method of investigating such women was by dilatation and curettage (D&C), a blind sampling technique performed under general anaesthesia with a sharp metal curette. Hysteroscopy, the direct visualisation of the uterine cavity with an endoscope, has superseded D&C[9] and will identify intrauterine pathologies in approximately 45% of this group of women. In other words, 55% of women investigated by hysteroscopy will have an apparently normal uterus (DUB).

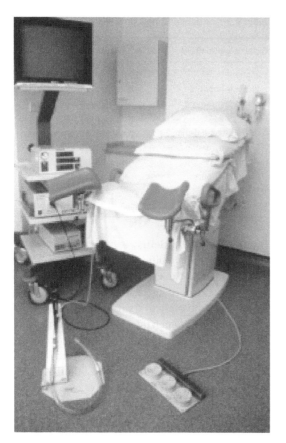

Figure 9.1 A typical outpatient hysteroscopy setting.

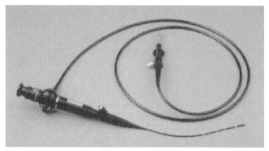

Figure 9.2 A typical flexible hysteroscope.

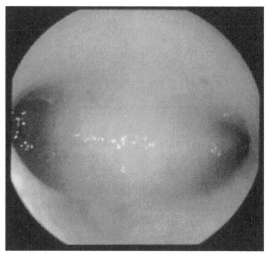

Figure 9.3 Hysteroscopic view of a normal uterine cavity.

With the advances in lens technology, hystero-scopes have become smaller and more versatile and are now routinely used in the outpatient setting with no analgesia required.[10–12] Figure 9.1 shows a standard outpatient hysteroscopy set-up with the chair, and camera stack allowing the patient to watch the hysteroscopy if she wishes. Figure 9.2 shows a standard flexible hysteroscope routinely used in the outpatient setting.

As so many women were found to have normal uterine cavities (Fig. 9.3), this led to the recent inter-est in transvaginal ultrasound as a screening tool for the diagnosis of normality in such women. The advantages are that it is a non-invasive procedure and more realistic use of resources.

If normality can be used as the basis for screening with ultrasound, why can ultrasound not be used for all cases of AUB in premenopausal women? The limi-tation of ultrasound in the presence of pathology is its inability to define the presence, location and character of any given abnormality reliably. The sen-sitivity of transvaginal ultrasound in this situation is at best 75%.[13,14] Studies that have assessed the role of ultrasound in such a group of women have failed to justify its place in clinical practice because of the need for the clinician to be able to map the abnormality accurately, so that appropriate treat-ment may be provided.[15]

At present, therefore, ultrasound has a potential role in acting as a triage mechanism in women with DUB by screening out those patients who do not require subsequent hysteroscopy. There may be additional benefit in the use of ultrasound in this group of women because of the ability to visualise the ovaries. Whether additional information on ovarian pathology, gathered during the ultrasound, is a bonus, has yet to be clarified.

Management of dysfunctional uterine bleeding

The management of patients in whom no intrauterine pathology is discovered at investigation can be through either medical or surgical therapy. Medical therapy consists of hormonal-based or non-hormonally based drugs. If the menstrual cycle is chaotic, progesterone is often used to stabilise the menstrual loss. Alternatively, if there are no contraindications, the combined oral contraceptive pill is excellent in controlling menstrual loss, especially in a younger woman who also requires contraception. In a non-smoking patient the pill can be used beyond the age of 35. Non-hormonal therapy acts by controlling the haemostatic mechanisms in the endometrium, for example, tranexamic acid, or the prostaglandin production in the uterus, for example, mefenamic acid. Mefenamic acid is used in women who have a regular but heavy menstrual loss and is taken only whilst the woman is menstruating.

The Mirena intrauterine system

A more recent development, the Mirena intrauterine system (IUS), licensed in the UK in May 1995, was initially marketed as a contraceptive device but over the last decade it has become a very versatile treatment option for a variety of clinical indications and it is now used widely throughout the UK. Potential uses of the Mirena IUS include:

- contraception
- fibroids
- premens trial syndrome
- hormone replacement therapy
- endometrial hyperplasia
- endometriosis
- adenomyosis

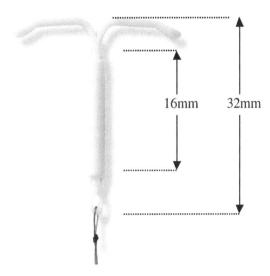

Figure 9.4 The Mirena intrauterine system.

- tamoxifen users
- endometrial preparation
- menorrhagia

The Mirena IUS (Fig. 9.4) comprises a T-shaped polyethylene frame carrying a white hormone cylinder 19 mm in length around the vertical arm, creating an outer diameter of 2.8 mm. The cylinder contains a mixture of polydimethylsiloxane (50%) and levonorgestrel (LNG) (50%) and is covered by a polydimethylsiloxane membrane, which regulates the release of the LNG. The total amount of LNG in the system is 52 mg. After insertion into the uterus, LNG is released from the reservoir at an initial rate of 20 µg/24 hours directly to the endometrium. The T-shaped frame is impregnated with barium sulphate to make the system X-ray-detectable. Dark monofilament polyethylene threads are attached to the lower end of the vertical arm.

The Mirena may be left in situ for 5 years. The therapeutic effects of the Mirena IUS are based on local effects in the uterus. The progesterone release has a contraceptive action that complements the mechanical effect of the device but it also has a direct effect on the function of the adjacent endometrium. Endometrial proliferation has been shown to be prevented by the local administration of LNG, which inhibits the function of oestradiol in the endometrium;[16] also LNG thickens the cervical mucus, thus inhibiting sperm motility and function.[17] Suppression of ovulation may occur in some women using the Mirena IUS, but on average 75% of cycles have been shown to be ovulatory.[17,18] The device may also have a weak foreign-body effect.[16]

Patients presenting with menorrhagia whose symptoms are refractory to conventional medical therapy traditionally face the choice of either undergoing a hysterectomy or, more recently, alternative, less invasive surgical treatment. Endometrial resection is the alternative to hysterectomy that has been formally assessed in clinical trials.[19–22] This involves a general anaesthetic, insertion of an operative hysteroscope and the removal of the endometrial lining using a loop through which diathermy is passed cutting through and destroying the endometrium. The benefits to the patient include shorter hospital stay, less postoperative morbidity, quicker return to work and speedier overall recovery.

More recently, newer second-generation ablative techniques[23] have increased in both number and popularity, having been developed to equal or exceed the efficacy of the first-generation ablative methods, whilst simultaneously aiming to reduce the complications by removing the requirement for hysteroscopic skills. The intention is for the newer technologies to be suitable for use by general gynaecologists who will not have undergone the lengthy training necessary for endometrial resection. These techniques use ablative methods such as microwave and circulation of hot water in balloons. These techniques, unlike the traditional resection method, are blind and therefore a request for ultrasound may be made to assess the thinnest part of the uterine wall to evaluate the risk of uterine perforation during the procedure.

Hysterectomy is the most traditional surgical method and can be performed by the abdominal route (usually with a transverse scar in the lower abdomen) or by the vaginal route. The reason for using the abdominal route as opposed to the vaginal route was often because of operator preference,

uterine size or the presence of other pelvic pathology, such as adhesions and ovarian cysts. With the introduction of laparoscopic-assisted vaginal hysterectomy (LAVH), the ability to perform a vaginal hysterectomy in more cases is now possible.

Premenopausal abnormal uterine bleeding – key points

- Hysteroscopy identifies pathology in about 45% of women
- 55% have dysfunctional uterine bleeding with no evident pathology
- Ultrasound:
  - is a useful screening tool, identifying pathology such as polyps or fibroids
  - screens out those with a normal uterus who would otherwise have gone on to hysteroscopy
  - is limited in its ability to map the location of abnormalities accurately and reliably characterise them
  - may give useful additional information regarding the ovaries
- Treatment options for dysfunctional uterine bleeding include:
  - medical therapy
  - Mirena intrauterine system
  - endometrial resection – traditional or second-generation
  - hysterectomy

Postmenopausal patients

Women with PMB are often anxious about the possibility of cancer and frequently concerned about the need for an operation. Investigations in this group of women should aim to exclude serious pathology but should also use the investigation to give the woman the maximum amount of information to help make decisions when choosing management.

Women with abnormal bleeding after the menopause are a group more at risk of endometrial cancer than their premenopausal counterparts. The risk of cancer increases with age; therefore there is a need for more urgent investigation in this group of patients. Once more, the traditional approach to investigation was by performing a D&C but latterly hysteroscopy has taken over as the gold standard. If ultrasound is used as the screening tool in this group it is essential that its accuracy in excluding pathology matches that of direct visualisation at hysteroscopy, especially as hysteroscopy, as an outpatient procedure, has become more patient-acceptable.[24] Attempts at utilising ultrasound in PMB patients have centred on the measurement of endometrial thickness. It has been suggested that an endometrial thickness of less than 5 mm is a useful screening end-point for the determination of normality.[25] Many studies have taken other measurements (< 3 and < 4 mm).[26] There are a number of problems with this approach: firstly, endometrial cancers have been identified in women whose endometrium is less than 5 mm.[27] This may mean that a lower cut-off measurement should be used, but this would then generate an increased number of hysteroscopies. Secondly, there is considerable intra- and interobserver variation in ultrasound measurements, which would have to be taken into account if universal screening becomes employed.[28]

The same arguments concerning the identification of abnormalities in premenopausal women apply to postmenopausal women. The latter are still likely to have endometrial polyps (22%) and fibroids (15%). In addition, the presence of endometrial hyperplasia (a pathological diagnosis with a risk of coincident endometrial cancer which may be found as a localised area of thickened endometrium) may be missed.

In both these categories of patients there are continuing developments in ultrasound technology that show promise in improving diagnostic accuracy. The use of a contrast medium, in the form of saline, appears to enhance the view obtained, allowing accurate visualisation of polyps and fibroids. In addition, the saline may make the definition of a thin endometrium easier. Doppler studies of the endometrial–myometrial interface to identify vascular angiogenesis have looked promising[29] but have not been widely adopted in routine practice. How-

ever the detection of feeding vessels with Doppler has been useful in identifying polyps.

Postmenopausal bleeding and tamoxifen

A specific group of postmenopausal patients is attracting an increasing number of new referrals to gynaecologists and ultrasonographers. This group consists of patients with breast cancer who are on long-term tamoxifen therapy. Tamoxifen, which is a partial oestrogen antagonist, is extremely effective in controlling breast disease. Its antagonistic action, however, is in the endometrium. This can lead to excessive oestrogen stimulation in the endometrium and endometrial polyps, endometrial proliferation and, in some cases, endometrial cancer. The exact relationship between tamoxifen and its endometrial effects is currently being investigated. Tamoxifen-related polyps and endometrial changes may be difficult to detect by ultrasound. Because of the tissue effects of tamoxifen, the endometrium can simply seem thickened, but when subsequent hysteroscopy is carried out the true nature of the lesion is seen. The polyps are often very soft and vascular with stromal thickening and oedema, and their removal is essential.

Postmenopausal abnormal uterine bleeding – key points

- This group has an increased risk of endometrial carcinoma
- Hysteroscopy is the gold standard for investigation
- Ultrasound:
  - can be used as a screening tool
  - enables measurement of the endometrial thickness, which correlates with the presence of pathology
  - the cut-off point, in millimetres, is a balance between generating too many hysteroscopies (if set too low) and missing abnormalities (if set too high)
  - Tamoxifen may be associated with endometrial proliferation, polyps and endometrial cancer

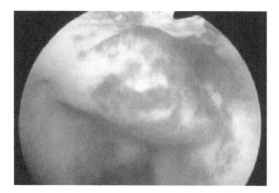

Figure 9.5 Hysteroscopic view of an endometrial polyp.

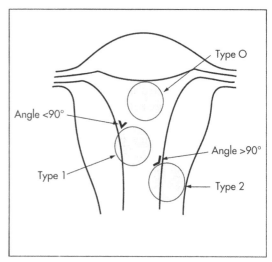

Figure 9.7 Classification of submucous fibroids. Courtesy of the European Society of Hysteroscopy.

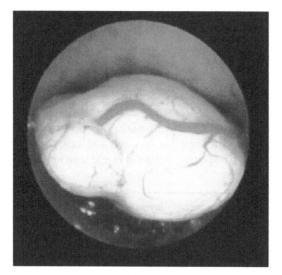

Figure 9.6 Hysteroscopic view of a fibroid (type 0).

Fibroids and polyps

In both groups of patients with AUB, fibroids and polyps can be found at hysteroscopy and ultrasound. From the clinical viewpoint, the exact site and character of these lesions are becoming important issues. There is a growing body of evidence that the removal of the lesion alone, rather than the total removal of the uterus, has a successful chance of improving the patient's symptoms.[30,31] With advances in hysteroscopic surgery it is now possible to remove these lesions with the minimum of trauma and under direct vision.

Polyps (Fig. 9.5) are exuberant endometrial proliferation and, more often than not, are benign in nature. However, they can be the site of endometrial carcinoma and as such should be removed in postmenopausal women.[32] Removal of polyps in symptomatic women is more likely to result in cessation of symptoms in the postmenopausal group than the premenopausal group. The difficulty ultrasound has in the detection of polyps is in differentiating between a thick endometrium and that containing a polyp.

Fibroids can be found in three places in the uterus. They may be subserosal, on the outer surface of the uterus, intramural, within the myometrial wall, or submucous, impinging on the endometrial cavity (Fig. 9.6). The former is not amenable to hysteroscopic surgery and is also unlikely to be involved in the evolution of the patient's bleeding symptoms. Fibroids in the intramural portion of the uterus may be removed by hysteroscopic resection, but it is difficult. The final site, impinging on the endometrial cavity, is the site most amenable to hysteroscopic surgery.[30] For the patient and the clinician, it is important to know the exact site of the submucous fibroid (Fig. 9.7). How much of the fibroid is present in the endometrial cavity as opposed to the wall of the uterus and the size of the fibroid are important pieces of information. Both these issues are taken into account during patient counselling and are indices used to establish the ability to treat. The success rate of the procedure is also determined, preoperatively, using these indices. Patients need to be warned of the possibility of a two-stage procedure to treat the fibroid and this can only be done if the information is available. To date, hysteroscopy is the best way of obtaining this information but contrast sonography may prove useful in the future.

Fibroids and polyps – key points

- Treatment options for fibroids include hysteroscopic resection or hysterectomy
- Submucous fibroids are more amenable to hysteroscopic removal than intramural fibroids. The exact location and size of the lesion are important in treatment planning, counselling and in predicting the success of treatment
- Polyps may be the site of endometrial carcinoma
- Removal of polyps alleviates symptoms in postmenopausal women more successfully than in premenopausal women

---

Pelvic masses and gynaecological cancer

Patients are often referred specifically to investigate a pelvic mass. The most serious concern is that of ovarian carcinoma. Other reasons for a pelvic mass are large fibroids, benign ovarian cysts, inflammatory masses and non-gynaecological causes (such as inflammatory bowel disease, diverticular disease and colonic carcinoma). Usually, the patient's symptoms are not overt but, occasionally, there are vague symptoms of abdominal bloatedness or pressure symptoms relating to bladder function.

Ultrasound plays a key role in the differentiation of pelvic masses. Large fibroids are usually readily identifiable. If not removed surgically by the clinician, subsequent monitoring of the fibroid can be performed with further ultrasound scans in order to assess pressure on the renal tract and subsequent hydronephrosis. Ovarian cysts can be easily identified by ultrasound. Features suggestive, but not indicative, of malignancy are solid and cystic components and vascular neogenesis as seen with Doppler examination.[33] Usually, laparotomy is carried out in the presence of a suspicious pelvic mass and the final histology is obtained thereafter. Subsequent follow-up of patients with malignant disease of the ovary may occasionally be carried out by ultrasound, but CT is superior in its ability to stage and monitor spread of disease.

Malignant ovarian tumours

Malignant ovarian cysts all need to be removed at laparotomy. The nature of ovarian cancer is that it tends to present late in the stage of the disease, and this often means that the disease has spread beyond the pelvis. Computed tomography (CT) is superior to ultrasound in its ability to stage the disease, detecting spread into adjacent organs, omentum and lymphadenopathy. It provides a good baseline for monitoring the results of debulking surgery and the effects of subsequent chemotherapy.

Surgery for ovarian cancer necessitates removal of as much of the malignancy as possible and usually means a hysterectomy, removal of both ovaries and, in addition, removal of the omentum and appendix. The ability of postoperative chemotherapy, as needed in nearly all cases, to be effective, is to some extent determined by the volume of disease remaining after surgery. The smaller the volume of tissue, the better the chance of a response. The prognosis for ovarian cancer also depends on the stage of the disease; the more confined the cancer, the better the outcome. Despite this, because of the late presentation of the disease in many women, the overall survival for ovarian cancer is poor. The cumulative lifetime risk of developing ovarian cancer is 1.5% and the risk of dying from cancer is similar, 1.3%.

Benign ovarian tumours

Ovarian masses that appear benign and are persistently greater than 4 cm in diameter may need to be explored surgically with subsequent removal. If left in place ovarian cysts may bleed or tort and can therefore result in an acute episode with emergency admission. It is better to have the cyst removed electively. Benign ovarian cysts can often be removed laparoscopically, but sometimes there is no normal remaining tissue and in these cases the whole ovary may need to be removed together with the cyst.

Benign ovarian cysts are more likely to be unilocular and completely cystic. Physiological benign cysts, such as ovulatory cysts and corpus luteal cysts, are well recognised and, if doubt exists, may be rescanned at a different stage in the cycle to ensure resolution. Usually, cysts fewer than 4 cm in diameter resolve spontaneously.

Dermoid cysts are benign cystic teratomas and have solid features within the cyst. As there is the chance of bilateral dermoid cysts in a proportion of patients, screening of the non-affected ovary is important. Occult cysts, seen at ultrasound in the presumed unaffected ovary, would warrant a careful examination at the time of removal of the affected side.

Ovarian fibromas are benign, hard, solid tumours which generally carry no risk of malignancy. These may be found incidentally, most frequently around 50 years of age, and fewer than 10% of cases are bilateral. Most can be managed conservatively. However, surgical removal may be necessary if the lesions are large, causing symptoms, or in rare cases of Meigs' syndrome (1% of cases) when they cause ascites and pleural effusions.

Ovarian screening

Screening for ovarian cancer by ultrasound has been investigated.[34] Pelvic ultrasound in combination with CA125 (a tumour marker) has been the method used (see chapter 6). However, if this screening procedure was introduced in the general population, a huge number of people would have to be screened to detect a very small number of malignancies. In addition, a substantial number of patients would have benign cysts and would undergo laparotomy for a non-malignant condition. Overall, this strategy for screening has not been pursued because

of the above considerations. In high-risk families, who have a first-degree or close relative with ovarian cancer, limited screening is available. It is important that this screening is done in a facility where genetic counselling is available.

Cervical cancer

Cervical cancer tends to be diagnosed clinically or as a result of cervical cytology. However ultrasound, may be important in the preliminary investigation of patients. If ureteral involvement is suspected identification of ureteral dilatation or pelvicalyceal dilatation would then lead to more extensive investigation using CT.

Pelvic masses – key points

- Pelvic masses may present with abdominal bloating and/or bladder symptoms
- Ultrasound is the first-line investigation
- Treatment options for ovarian carcinoma include:
  - computed tomography for staging of carcinoma and postoperative follow-up
  - laparotomy-hysterectomy, bilateral salpingo-oophorectomy, omentectomy and lymphadenectomy
  - postoperative chemotherapy.
- Diagnosis of cervical cancer is usually made clinically and with cervical cytology. Ultrasound may identify renal tract involvement

---

Infertility

This is comprehensively discussed in Chapter 7.

Investigation of the infertile couple

In routine clinical practice there are three areas causing problems with conception: (1) male factor; (2) tubal factor; and (3) anovulation. A semen analysis should be obtained from all couples before any invasive investigations are performed on the female partner to establish or exclude male-factor infertility. Tubal disease is best assessed by laparoscopy and dye test, hysterosalpingography or hystero-contrast sonography.[35] The diagnosis of anovulation is usually made by repeat progesterone assays around day 21 of a 28-day cycle. Causes of anovulation, such as polycystic ovaries, can be readily identified by ultrasound and characteristic features recognised.[36]

In women with long menstrual cycles, timing by dates may be impossible, and in these cases follicular mapping, performed serially, can be very useful in determining the correct time to carry out the test and to time intercourse.

Monitoring of assisted conception

Ultrasound monitoring of ovarian and endometrial response to stimulation regimes is now established practice in fertility centres. The ability to time cycles, harvest eggs and to prevent multiple pregnancies has been made possible by the concomitant use of ultrasound and hormonal monitoring, and it is essential for the guidance of harvest procedures, obviating the need for laparoscopic egg retrieval.[37]

Ultrasound is also useful in reducing the complications associated with therapy. Ovarian hyperstimulation, following the maturation of a large number of follicles, is one of the most serious complications for women undergoing gonadotrophin therapy, and is responsible for major maternal morbidity. The underlying problem of capillary leakage from the stimulated ovary can lead to ascites, pleural effusions, hypovolaemia and venous thrombosis. The problem can be avoided or reduced by withholding administration of the ovulation induction agent (human chorionic gonadotrophin) when too many follicles are present.[38]

Endometriosis

Endometriosis is defined as the presence of tissue that is histologically similar to endometrium outside the uterine cavity and the myometrium. It is a relatively common disease with estimates from 2 to 50% of all women who undergo laparoscopy.

The relationship between endometrosis and infertility is complex and poorly understood. The prevalence within the infertile population is between 20 and 40%. The main symptoms are dysmenorrhoea, pelvic pain, dyspareunia and infertility.

The use of transvaginal ultrasound has improved the diagnosis of clinically undetectable ovarian cysts but it has a poor sensitivity.

The wide range of presentations of endometriosis allows a variety of treatment options to be considered depending on age, need for contraception, reproductive status and so on. The main goals of treatment are to relieve symptoms and restore fertility where necessary. Treatment includes medical options such as the combined oral contraceptive pill, progestogens, danazol and gonadotrophin-releasing hormone analogues. Surgical options include laparoscopic diathermy to endometriosis, excision, ovarian cystectomy or hysterectomy and oophorectomy.

The acute pelvis

Female patients admitted via casualty with a history of acute lower abdominal pain are often assessed by gynaecologists. The first diagnosis to exclude or consider is ectopic pregnancy, which is discussed under pregnancy-related gynaecological conditions, below.

Pelvic inflammatory disease

The second most common condition to consider is pelvic inflammatory disease. The symptoms most often described in pelvic infection are bilateral low abdominal pain and a vaginal discharge. Patients are not always pyrexial. Examination usually reveals bilateral iliac fossa tenderness, sometimes with guarding, with both adnexal regions usually tender to palpation. Vaginal examination may reveal a cervical discharge, but not always. The diagnosis is based on the clinical symptoms and confirmatory bacterial swabs; however, ultrasound can be used to corroborate the findings and, more usefully, to exclude other pathology. The finding of fluid in the pouch of Douglas has been used to help confirm a clinical suspicion of pelvic inflammatory disease[39] but may also be found in a ruptured ectopic pregnancy. A pelvic abscess has characteristic appearances on ultrasound and the patient is often quite toxic.

Patients with a suspected diagnosis of pelvic inflammatory disease are usually treated with antibiotics, after bacterial swabs have been taken from the endocervix and the high vagina. Registration with a genitourinary clinic with contact tracing is also an important part of the patient's management. Occasionally, if the patient's symptoms do not respond to conservative antibiotic therapy, a diagnostic laparoscopy is carried out to ensure there is no pelvic collection or abscess formation. In patients with a pelvic abscess, intravenous antibiotics are also important but the abscess should be drained surgically at laparoscopy or via ultrasound guidance where amenable, in order for symptoms to resolve.

Ovarian cyst accidents

Pain low in the pelvis may also be associated with ovarian cysts. The commonest cysts to cause such symptoms are corpus luteal cysts, which have ruptured, usually postcoitally. Ovarian cysts may also become twisted on their pedicle (torted) or bleed internally into the substance of the cyst itself.

Patients who are admitted with a history of acute pelvic pain and who have a cyst diagnosed at subsequent ultrasound may need to undergo laparoscopy to assess the nature of the cyst and treat it accordingly if the pain does not settle with conservative management. Often a haemorrhagic cyst may require removal, together with the ovary, if it is affected. A torted ovarian cyst will need to be removed but the ovary may be conserved if it has not been affected by the interruption in its blood supply; in other words, if it has not become ischaemic. Laparoscopic treatment rather than laparotomy should be possible in the majority of cases.

Fibroid red degeneration

Pedunculated fibroids on the surface of the uterus can also be a source of pain because of torsion or red degeneration. The latter is most often associated with pregnancy and occurs as a result of the fibroid outgrowing its blood supply, with subsequent haemorrhage into itself. Fibroid red degeneration can be very difficult to manage, as the only option is pain relief until the pregnancy reaches a suitable gestation to deliver the baby.

The acute pelvis – key points

- High index of suspicion for ectopic pregnancy
- Pelvic inflammatory disease (PID) is a common cause of lower abdominal pain and may be accompanied by vaginal discharge
- Diagnosis of PID clinically is confirmed by bacterial swabs and ultrasound scan
- Treatment is with antibiotics and subsequent drainage of abscess if symptoms persist
- Ovarian cysts are assessed laparoscopically and may be removed if haemorrhagic or torted

---

Pregnancy-related gynaecological conditions

In most gynaecology units throughout the UK, the introduction of early-pregnancy assessment units has advanced the early diagnosis and management of complications of early pregnancy. Such units incorporate a dedicated team of nursing staff, familiar with early-pregnancy protocols, along with qualified ultrasonographers to perform the scanning. A multidisciplinary approach is recommended for the care of these women as it can obviously be a very difficult time, with uncertainty about the viability of their pregnancy.

Ectopic pregnancy

The incidence of ectopic pregnancy has shown a consistent increase during the last two or three decades, in particular with the increase in assisted conception techniques. However, it is difficult to compare the various publications because ectopic pregnancy is seldom described in absolute numbers. Most often it is expressed as an overall rate, such as ectopic pregnancy per 1000 live births. The current incidence rate for ectopic pregnancy in western societies is 11.5 per 1000 pregnancies. In the UK, ectopic pregnancy accounts for about 10% of maternal deaths and is the fifth commonest cause of direct maternal death.[40] In the western world as a whole, ectopic pregnancy is the major cause of maternal mortality in the first trimester.

Ectopic pregnancy is often difficult to diagnose and a high index of suspicion should be maintained when a woman of reproductive age complains of abdominal pain. In current practice, in patients with abdominal pain, the diagnosis is only definitive in fewer than 50% of cases. Ectopic pregnancy may mimic the symptoms of other gynaecological conditions, such as pelvic inflammatory disease, ruptured corpus luteum, DUB and incomplete abortion. Abdominal pain is the commonest symptom and is frequently present even before rupture. Amenorrhoea is reported in 75–95% of patients. The last menstrual period is often described as lighter than normal and may occur earlier or later than expected. The most common physical sign is abdominal tenderness, often associated with rebound tenderness.

The role of ultrasonography in suspected ectopic gestation is to attempt to localise the pregnancy. If the pregnancy is found to be intrauterine, ectopic pregnancy is virtually excluded because the combination of intrauterine and ectopic pregnancy is extremely rare in normal conceptions (1 in 30 000), although in stimulated in vitro fertilisation pregnancies the heterotopic pregnancy rate is higher. The interpretation of ultrasound findings is dependent on the accurate knowledge of the duration of amenorrhoea.

It is well known that more than a third of patients with ectopic pregnancy do not know the date of their last menstrual period, and in others irregular bleeding may lead to confusion. If no gestational sac or pregnancy is seen on transabdominal ultrasound and a pregnancy test is positive, an ectopic pregnancy is highly likely.

A major advantage of transvaginal sonography is that it can diagnose normal or failed intrauterine pregnancy at least 1 week earlier than by transabdominal sonography.[41] In particular, when trying to differentiate between a pseudogestational sac, as occurs with ectopic pregnancy, and a normal early intrauterine gestational sac, the transvaginal probe is more useful than a transabdominal scan.

Ectopic pregnancy is a potentially dangerous condition that should be managed with the utmost

of care. Initial expectant management with beta-human chorionic gonadotrophin monitoring is possible in women who are haemodynamically stable and where there is the possibility that the pregnancy is situated in the uterus. There are guidelines for this approach; when a suboptimal rise in the pregnancy hormone occurs the patient should undergo a diagnostic laparoscopy.

At laparoscopy the ectopic pregnancy can either be removed on its own after opening the fallopian tube (salpingostomy) or by removing of the ectopic and the fallopian tube (salpingectomy). Some centres are injecting the ectopic with methotrexate or hyperosmolar glucose to kill the pregnancy, and this may prove useful in the future. Most surgery should now be carried out laparoscopically with a reduction in postoperative pain and earlier recovery rates than when surgery is performed by laparotomy.

Cystic adnexal masses and free fluid in the pouch of Douglas are other sonographic signs which should raise the index of suspicion of the presence of a possible ectopic gestation. However, it is very difficult to differentiate between the other numerous possible underlying conditions such as pelvic inflammatory disease, ovarian cysts and endometriosis, all of which may mimic an ectopic pregnancy. In addition, it has been reported that the adnexal mass, as seen ultrasonically, can be on the contralateral side of the ectopic pregnancy in about 30% of cases, and normal adnexal findings on ultrasound have been seen in 20% of women with laparoscopically confirmed ectopic pregnancy. Overall, the use of sonography as a diagnostic test in suspected ectopic pregnancy allows an accurate diagnosis as to the presence or absence of an ectopic gestation in approximately 70–90% of affected cases.

Miscarriage

Bleeding in early pregnancy is a considerable source of distress to the patient. The concerns regarding the continuing viability of a pregnancy are very real and should be allayed as soon as possible. In the past, bleeding, was often a reason for immediate admission to a gynaecological ward but, with the introduction of early-pregnancy assessment units (EPAU) throughout the UK, the management is now carried out in outpatients. Ultrasound availability has played a critical role in the development of these units. Patients and general practitioners can now, at short notice, have an assessment of the uterus in the event of bleeding. Ultrasound helps clarify whether a pregnancy is ongoing or not.

Types of miscarriage vary, and can be categorised on history, examination and ultrasound findings. A complete miscarriage means the conception has been lost completely. The patient will often have a history of heavy bleeding with clots followed by crampy abdominal pain with subsequent reduction in both the vaginal loss and pain. On ultrasound the uterus should be empty. In cases of incomplete miscarriage, ultrasound will identify remaining products of conception. A missed miscarriage, where the pregnancy has stopped developing and only the gestational sac remains, also has a characteristic appearance.

Trophoblastic disease

Occasionally a pregnancy which has become complicated by excessive trophoblastic proliferation is picked up at a routine pregnancy scan in the first trimester. These molar pregnancies can be easily treated by evacuation of the uterus and, occasionally, methotrexate therapy. The classical appearances on ultrasound are of an enlarged uterus filled with echogenic material in the early stages, developing easily visible cystic vesicles as the mole progresses, which considerably increases through transmission of the beam. There are a handful of centres throughout the UK that follow up all patients with molar pregnancies and maintain a national database. They monitor the urinary beta-human chorionic gonadotrophin levels to ensure they return to normal levels and do not proceed to chorionic carcinoma.

In women who miscarry recurrently (defined as more than three times) the early ultrasound findings of a normally situated and viable pregnancy provide the woman with a 95% chance of an eventual good outcome. The reassurance value of such a non-invasive intervention early in pregnancy is significant. A randomised trial of early scanning and active reassurance found a significant benefit, in terms of pregnancy outcome, to those women who received supportive care by scanning and reassurance compared with those who did not.[42]

The future

The quality and definition of ultrasound technology are improving all the time. As our understanding increases, the scope for incorporation into clinical practice will inevitably improve. Saline infusion hysterosonography (SIH) is a concept attracting increasingly innovative practice with obvious clinical usefulness. Saline is infused into the uterine cavity to enhance visualisation of its contents during a transvaginal ultrasound examination.[43–50] Although initially used to investigate tubal patency,[51] SIH rapidly evolved into an investigation of the uterine cavity. The advantage of SIH is that it is relatively non-invasive compared to hysteroscopy, it is performed during transvaginal ultrasound and it can therefore also identify ovarian pathology.[52]

The use of ultrasound is also likely to become increasingly established as a guidance mechanism for minimally invasive therapies, increasing patient choices and improving gynaecological management.

REFERENCES

1. I. Donald, Use of ultrasonics in the diagnosis of abdominal swelling. *British Medical Journal*, **2** (1963), 1154–5.

2. J. MacVicar and I. Donald, Sonar in the diagnosis of early pregnancy and its complications. *Journal of Obstetrics and Gynaecology of the British Commmwealth*, **70** (1963), 387–95.

3. H. P. Robinson, Sonar in the puerperium, a means of diagnosing retained products of conception. *Scottish Medical Journal*, **17** (1972), 364–6.

4. A. Kratochwil, Ein neues vaginales Schnittbildverfahren. *Geburtshilfe Frauenheilkd*, **29** (1969), 379–85.

5. S. R. Schwimer and J. Lebovic, Transvaginal pelvic ultrasonography: accuracy in follicle and cyst size determination. *Journal of Ultrasound in Medicine*, **4** (1985), 61–3.

6. S. R. Goldstein, J. R. Snyder, C. Watson and M. Danon, Very early pregnancy detection with endovaginal ultrasound. *Obstetrics and Gynecology*, **72** (1988), 200–4.

7. A. Rempen, Vaginal sonography in ectopic pregnancy: a prospective evaluation. *Journal of Ultrasound in Medicine*, **7** (1987), 381–7.

8. Y. C. Choo, K. C. Mak, C. Hsu, T. S. Wong and H. K. Ma, Postmenopausal uterine bleeding of non organic cause. *Obstetrics and Gynecology*, **66** (1985), 225–8.

9. M. H. Goldrath and A. I. Sherman, Office hysteroscopy and suction curettage: can we eliminate the hospital diagnostic dilatation and curettage? *American Journal of Obstetrics and Gynecology*, **152** (1985), 220–9.

10. L Rogerson and S. Duffy, National survey of outpatient hysteroscopy. *Gynaecology and Endoscopy*, **10** (2001), 343–7.

11. C. Kremer, S. Barik and S. Duffy, Flexible outpatient hysteroscopy without anaesthesia: a safe, successful and well tolerated procedure. *British Journal of Obstetrics and Gynaecology*, **105** (1998), 672–6.

12. C. Kremer, S. Duffy and M. Moroney, Patient satisfaction with outpatient hysteroscopy versus day case hysteroscopy: randomised controlled trial. *British Medical Journal*, **320** (2000), 279–82.

13. B. Cacciatore, T. Ramsay, P. Lehtovirta and P. Ylostalo, Transvaginal sonography and hysteroscopy in postmenopausal bleeding. *Acta Obstetrica Gynecologica Scandinavica*, **73** (1994), 413–16.

14. Z. Weiner, D. Beck, S. Rottem, J. Brandes and I. Thaler, Uterine artery flow velocity waveforms and color flow imaging in women with perimenopausal and postmenopausal bleeding. *Acta Obstetrica Gynecologica Scandinavica*, **72** (1993), 162–6.

15. E. Cicinelli, F. Romano, P. S. Anastasio, *et al.* Transabdominal sonohysterography, transvaginal sonography, and hysteroscopy in the evaluation of submucous myomas. *Obstetrica Gynecologica*, **85** (1995), 42–7.

16. S. G. Silverberg, M. Haukkamaa, H. Arko, C. G. Nilsson and T. Luukkainen, Endometrial morphology during long-term use of levonorgestrel-releasing intrauterine devices. *International Journal of Gynecological Pathology*, **5** (1986), 235–41.

17. I. Barbosa, O. Bakos, S. E. Olsson, V. Odlind and E. D. B. Johansson, Ovarian function during use of a levonorgestrel-releasing IUD. *Contraception*, **42** (1990), 51–66.

18. C. G. Nilsson, P. Lahteenmaki and T. Luukkainen, Ovarian function in amenorrhoeic and menstruating users of a levonorgestrel-releasing intrauterine device. *Fertility and Sterility*, **41** (1984), 52–5.

19. M. J. Gannon, E. M. Holt, J. Fairbank *et al.*, A randomised controlled trial comparing endometrial resection and abdominal hysterectomy for the treatment of menorrhagia. *British Medical Journal*, **303** (1991), 1362–4.

20. N. Dwyer, J. Hutton and G. M. Stirrat, Randomised controlled trial comparing endometrial resection with abdominal hysterectomy for the surgical treatment of menorrhagia. *British Journal of Obstetrics and Gynaecology*, **100** (1993), 237–43

21. S. B. Pinion, D. E. Parkin, D. R. Abramovich *et al.*, Randomised controlled trial of hysterectomy, endometrial laser ablation, and transcervical resection for dysfunctional uterine bleeding. *British Medical Journal*, **309** (1994), 979–83.

22. H. O'Connor, J. A. M. Broadbent, A. Magos and K. McPherson, Medical Research Council randomised controlled trial of endometrial resection versus hysterectomy in management of menorrhagia. *Lancet*, **349** (1997), 897–901.

23. C. Kremer and S. D. Duffy, Endometrial ablation: the next generation. *British Journal of Obstetrics and Gynaecology*, **107** (2000), 1443–52.

24. F. Nagele, H. O'Connor, A. Davies, *et al.*, 2500 outpatient diagnostic hysteroscopies. *Obstetrics and Gynecology*, **88** (1996), 87–92.

25. M. N. Nasri, J.H. Shepherd, M.E. Setchell, D.G. Lowe and T. Chard, The role of vaginal scan in measurement of endometrial thickness in postmenopausal women. *British Journal of Obstetrics and Gynaecology*, **98** (1991), 470–5.

26. S. Granberg, M. Wikland, B. Karlsson, A. Norstrom and L. Friberg, Endometrial thickness as measured by endovaginal ultrasonography for identifying endometrial abnormality. *American Journal of Obstetrics and Gynecology*, **164** (1991), 47–52.

27. A. Dorum, B. Kristensen, A. Langebrekke, T. Sornes and O. Skaar, Evaluation of endometrial thickness measured by endovaginal ultrasound in women with postmenopausal bleeding. *Acta Obstetrica Gynecologica Scandinavica*, **72** (1993), 116–19.

28. B. Karlsson, S. Granberg, B. Ridell and M. Wikland, Endometrial thickness as measured by transvaginal sonography: interobserver variation. *Ultrasound in Obstetrics and Gynecology*, **4** (1994), 320–5.

29. T. H. Bourne, S. Campbell, C. V. Steer *et al.*, Detection of endometrial cancer by transvaginal ultrasonography with color flow imaging and blood flow analysis: a preliminary report. *Gynecology and Oncology*, **40** (1991), 253–9.

30. S. G. Derman, J. Rehnstrom and R. S. Neuwirth, The long-term effectiveness of hysteroscopic treatment of menorrha-

gia and leiomyomas. *Obstetrics and Gynecology*, **4** (1991), 591–4.

31. K. Wamsteker, M. H. Emanuel and J. H. De Kruif, Transcervical hysteroscopic resection of submucous fibroids for abnormal uterine bleeding: results regarding the degree of intramural extension. *Obstetrics and Gynecology*, **82** (1993), 736–40.

32. B. Petterson, H. O. Adami, A. Lindgren and I. Hesselius, Endometrial polyps and hyperplasia as risk factors for endometrial carcinoma. *Acta Obstetrica Gynecologica Scandinavica*, **64** (1985), 653–9.

33. U. J. Herrmann, G. W. Locher and A. Goldhirsch, Sonographic patterns of ovarian tumours. Prediction of malignancy. *Obstetrics and Gynecology*, **69** (1987), 777–81.

34. M. J. Webb, Screening for ovarian cancer. Still a long way to go. *British Medical Journal*, **306** (1993), 1015–16.

35. S. Campbell, T. H. Bourne, S. L. Tan and W. P. Collins, Hysterosalpingo contrast sonography (hycosy) and its future role within the investigation of infertility in Europe. *Ultrasound in Obstetrics and Gynecology*, **4** (1994), 245–53.

36. A. H. Balen, J. S. E. Laven, S. L. Tan and D. Dewailly, Ultrasound assessment of the polycystic ovary: international consensus definitions. *Human Reproduction Update*, **9** (2003), 1–10.

37. P. Dellenbach, P. Nisand, L. Moreau *et al.*, Transvaginal sonographically controlled ovarian follicle puncture for egg retrieval. *Lancet*, **1** (1984), 1467.

38. P. R. Brinsden, I. Wada, S. L. Tan, A. Balen and H. S. Jacobs, Diagnosis, prevention and management of ovarian hyperstimulation syndrome. *British Journal of Obstetrics and Gynaecology*, **102** (1995), 767–72.

39. S. Kupesic, A. Kurjak, L. Pasalic, S. Benic and M. Ilijas, The value of transvaginal color Doppler in the assessment of pelvic inflammatory disease. *Ultrasound Medicine and Biology*, **21** (1995), 733–8.

40. Department of Health, *Why Mothers Die. Report on Confidential Enquiries into Maternal Deaths in the United Kingdom 1994–1996* (London: TSO, 1998).

41. I. Stabile and J. G. Grudzinskas, Ectopic pregnancy: what's new? In J. Studd, ed. *Progress in Obstetrics and Gynaecology*, vol. 11 (Edinburgh: Churchill Livingstone, 1995), pp. 281–309.

42. H. S. Liddell, N. S. Pattison and A. Zanderigo, Recurrent miscarriage – outcome after supportive care in early pregnancy. *Australia and New Zealand Journal of Obstetrics and Gynecology*, **31** (1991), 320–2.

43. J. Van Roessel, K. Wamstaker and N. Exalto, Sonographic investigation of the uterus during artificial uterine cavity distension. *Journal of Clinical Ultrasound*, **15** (1987), 439–50.

44. C. H. Syrop and V. Sahakain, Transvaginal sonographic detection of endometrial polyps with fluid contrast augmentation. *Obstetrics and Gynecology*, **79** (1992), 1041–3.

45. F. Bonilla-Munsoles, C. Simon, V. Serra, M. Sampaio and A. Pellicer, An assessment of hysterosalpingosonography (HSSG) as a diagnostic tool for uterine cavity defects and tubal patency. *Journal of Clinical Ultrasound*, **20** (1992), 175–81.

46. A. K. Parsons and J. J. Lense, Sonohysterography for endometrial abnormalities: preliminary results. *Journal of Clinical Ultrasound*, **21** (1993), 87–95.

47. J. R. Cohen, D. Luxman, J. Sagi *et al.*, Sonohysterography for distinguishing endometrial thickening from endometrial polyps in postmenopausal bleeding. *Ultrasound in Obstetrics and Gynecology*, **4** (1994), 227–80.

48. S. R. Goldstein, Use of ultrasonohysterography for triage of perimenopausal patients with unexplained uterine bleeding. *American Journal of Obstetrics and Gynecology*, **170** (1994), 565–70.

49. T. J. Dubinsky, H. R. Parvey, G. Gormaz, M. Curtis and N. Maklad, Transvaginal hysterosonography: comparison with biopsy in the evaluation of post-menopausal bleeding. *Journal of Ultrasound in Medicine*, **14** (1995), 887–93.

50. T. J. Dubinsky, H. R. Parvey, G. Gormaz and N. Maklad, Transvaginal hysterosonography in the evaluation of small endoluminal masses. *Journal of Ultrasound in Medicine*, **14** (1995), 1–6.

51. T. S. Richman, G. N. Viscomi, A. de Cherney, M. L. Polan and L. O. Alcebo, Fallopian tubal patency assessed by ultrasound following fluid injection. *Radiology*, **152** (1984), 507–10.

52. L. Rogerson, J. Bates, M. Weston and S. Duffy, Outpatient hysteroscopy versus saline infusion hydrosonography (SIH). *British Journal of Obstetrics and Gynaecology*, **109** (2002), 800–4.

Index

Note: page numbers in *italics* refer to figures and tables

Lightning Source UK Ltd.
Milton Keynes UK
UKOW07f0614160815

256953UK00004B/31/P